Premed Prep

Premed Prep

~

*Advice from a Medical School
Admissions Dean*

SUNNY NAKAE

Rutgers University Press
New Brunswick, Camden, and Newark, New Jersey, and London

Library of Congress Cataloging-in-Publication Data

Names: Nakae, Sunny, author.
Title: Premed prep : advice from a medical school admissions dean / Sunny Nakae.
Description: New Brunswick, Camden : Rutgers University Press, [2021] |
Includes bibliographical references and index.
Identifiers: LCCN 2020008923 | ISBN 9781978817227 (paperback) |
ISBN 9781978817234 (hardcover) | ISBN 9781978817241 (epub) |
ISBN 9781978817258 (mobi) | ISBN 9781978817265 (pdf)
Subjects: LCSH: Premedical education—United States. | Medical colleges—
United States—Admission. | Medical education—Vocational guidance—
United States.
Classification: LCC R838 .N36 2021 | DDC 610.71/173—dc23
LC record available at https://lccn.loc.gov/2020008923

A British Cataloging-in-Publication record for this book is available from the
British Library.

♾ The paper used in this publication meets the requirements of the
American National Standard for Information Sciences—Permanence of Paper
for Printed Library Materials, ANSI Z39.48-1992.

www.rutgersuniversitypress.org

Manufactured in the United States of America

For my family and all my students past, present, and future

Contents

Part IV: Support Team Advice

Part V: Gap Years and Reapplying

Preface

Every fall my Facebook friends look forward to my posts from "your friendly neighborhood admissions dean" about my adventures with applicants. Most of the time these posts are foibles and amusing stories, and occasionally they are heartwarming triumphs. My friends and former students love these posts and frequently comment about how much they look forward to them each year. A few years ago I posted about a really bad admissions essay. In the comments I was challenged by a friend to "actually tell premeds what to write" instead of just posting bad examples.

This personal challenge led to me write a blog for ReflectiveMedEd.org, which is run by the Loyola University Chicago Stritch School of Medicine's Department of Medical Education. The blog entitled, *Tough Love for Your Personal Statement: Advice from a Medical School Admissions Dean*,[1] was the top blog in 2017 and remains so these years later. Readers told me that they appreciated my perspective and that it was helpful in their preparation.

I have been teaching premedical preparation topics around the country at conferences and events for more than fifteen years. Whenever I present I use anecdotes and a "keep it real" style that hopefully makes learning about preparation accessible, engaging, and ultimately effective. When I advise applicants one-on-one, I am known as the dean that will support you 100 percent, but I also give it to you straight and tell you the truth. I know that there is a need for more down-to-earth advice about the process and elements of applying to medical school, and that is what I hope to provide in this book.

I have been working with aspiring student doctors since 2001. I have answered thousands of questions about preparation over the years. I have been an encourager, an advocate, a realist, a cheerleader, and a pragmatist for students on the journey to medical school. This book is a compilation of the most common questions and issues that I have encountered over the years. If you and I were sitting on my deck and I could impart to you some pearls I've gathered from experience, this book would be the script. I address common pitfalls and give you inside advice that you can't get anywhere else. I have gathered this advice through national committee service, professional networks, and the many students who have trusted me with their dreams over the years.

The premed journey can be nerve racking, competitive, anxiety provoking, and difficult. Students worry about how they will be viewed, mistakes they have made, and what they will do if things do not work out. I know there is a lot of bad advice out there that contributes to the stress. There are online forums that stoke terror in aspiring doctors daily! But there are also wonderful resources, advisers, and allies that can provide concrete help along the way.

My goal with this book is to shift the paradigm from "What do I need to do to get into medical school?" to "What kind of person do I need to be in order to become a physician?" Focusing on personal development rather than the acquisition of experiences changes the focus in an important way. A personal development approach creates space for authenticity and joy.

This book is my effort to distill advice for students that will hopefully make the journey better. Using stories from my experiences with students, I take readers on the other side of the admissions office door. Whether you are a first-time applicant, a reapplicant, a parent of an aspiring physician, a prehealth adviser, or a friend of an aspiring physician, there is practical advice here to support the journey.

All of the stories in this book have been fictionalized or adapted to protect the innocent and unwitting, but they are absolutely based on the real experiences I've had over the years with applicants and premedical students. My hope is that by the end of this book, readers will have greater understanding and insight about medical school admissions that will better inform their preparations and their quests to become physicians. Supportive team members reading this book will better understand how to help, when to help, and what not to do.

This book is organized into five sections. The first offers tips and advice that you should read before you begin the premed journey. It gives the big picture for starting strong in college. I cannot stress enough how many current premeds or medical students have told me that they wish they had known and been given this advice earlier in their journey. It is critical to know how you are going to be evaluated in the long term so that you can be savvy from the beginning.

The second section has tips for premed preparation. The premed years can be difficult and confusing, but they don't have to be! This section provides advice on focusing on the right areas of development. I discuss getting out of a checklist mentality and how to actually enjoy your preparation. You'll find out the secrets to gaining a competitive edge, and it's probably not what you think!

Section three is about the application process and how to manage it well. You will learn how to present yourself well to decision makers who will determine whether or not you get a seat. I spend a lot of time talking about professionalism, which can be a major pitfall. The stories in this section are cautionary tales! Section four is advice for your support team: family, friends, and advisers. I hear far too many stories about stressors from the very people you expect to help you. These folk need to understand what effective support looks like, so I included some advice for them, too.

Section five covers gap years and gives advice for reapplying and continually assessing whether you are on a path that works for you. Finally, I leave you with some parting words and simple steps for success in a career in medicine. The book is written assuming that you already know many of the basics for applying to medical school. If you don't, then check out my simple overview in the appendix.

I love working with students and witnessing their journeys as they become physicians. I have dedicated my life to diversity, access, and equity in medical education and healthcare. At this point in my career I don't have enough time to spend providing encouragement and advice for every aspiring student doctor I meet. My former students are serving as physician mentors and referring their advisees to me as well, which I love! My hope is that this book will serve the purpose of letting you experience what it would be like to have a long, honest personal visit with me. Maybe you'll laugh, maybe you'll groan, and hopefully you'll learn something new and important for the journey.

PART I

Getting a Solid Start

1

Premed Basics

"Be Quick, but Don't Hurry"

The prevailing advice I give about academic progress in premedical preparation is a quote from the great John Wooden, one of the most successful coaches in NCAA college basketball history: "Be quick, but don't hurry." This seems contradictory, but in fact it's not. Go as fast as you can without your speed compromising your performance. If you sacrifice performance for speed it will not pay off. If you are in a hurry, you might make mistakes and not perform your best. This will lead to having to spend extra time addressing deficits, and that does not actually help you in the long run. What is the point of graduating in four years with a 2.9 grade point average? You will just end up taking at least a year of postbaccalaureate courses to really show you are prepared. Better to be intentional about your pace from day one.

My second most salient piece of advice is this: Your grade point average (GPA) will NOT get you in, but it can keep you out. You absolutely must safeguard your GPA during this process. The GPA is like a token that unlocks consideration for admission. Think of it like a key that determines how much the door is open. A lower GPA does not necessarily mean you'll be excluded, but it will mean that the number of schools that will consider you will be fewer than if your GPA were higher.

Notice I said it opens the door to "consideration." Schools typically prioritize their candidates by GPA to varying degrees, at least initially. How much consideration you receive is usually preliminarily based on your numbers. Some schools that are holistic have a minimum threshold that you have to meet before holistic review happens. Even schools that consider postbaccalaureate applicants may have minimum undergraduate GPAs that all candidates have to meet before they consider your postbaccalaureate performance. Admissions practices vary across schools, and as a rule having a solid GPA always helps.

Know the Rules

Before you begin, it is critical that you know this important rule for the American Medical College Application Service (AMCAS),[1] the common application to allopathic (MD-granting) medical schools. Every course you have ever taken for college credit will appear on your AMCAS application. You cannot repeat courses to improve your GPA. If you take a biology course for four credits and you earn a D, and then you repeat that course and earn an A, AMCAS will average in four credits of D and four credits of A into your GPA. Your university most likely will *replace* the four credits of the D grade with the four credits of the A grade. This makes getting off to a strong start and taking charge of your premed course journey that much more important.

Withdrawals

Let's have real talk with this important fact—withdrawals are not good, but they are better than Fs or Ds. Fs and Ds do real damage to your academic record and are hard to make up over time. You should enter college knowing the important dates for registration and course management at your school. You should know the last drop date and add date for courses. Know the minimum credits you have to take each semester. Find out whether you can take a class pass/fail and what the deadline is to switch that option to a graded course. Most schools do not allow pass/fail courses for the premedical coursework, but pass/fail courses *do not* affect your

AMCAS GPA. If you are not sure if you can do well, you may wish to pursue a pass/fail option in order to preview the class if auditing is not allowed or if you need the credits for financial aid purposes. If you fail a pass/fail class, your GPA calculation in AMCAS will not be impacted, but it will be noted on the academic summary page. (Your academic standing with your school might be affected.) Know if you are allowed to audit and if there are fees for auditing. Know when the final allowable withdrawal date is. Be aware of the academic progress, tuition refund, and financial aid policies related to withdrawing or dropping classes.

If something happens during the semester and you know you will not be able to earn at least a C, consider withdrawing and taking the W instead of a very poor grade. This is not to be taken lightly, of course, because a persistent pattern of withdrawals can be concerning for committees. Withdrawals also mean that you likely paid for the class and will have to do so again. Schools do not want to see someone continually withdrawing for fear of not getting perfect grades! But believe me, a W or two on the transcript will not affect your GPA, and you will live to tell the tale. You may still have to explain what happened during your interview, but you will be more likely to reach the interview phase of applying, rather than losing consideration because your GPA has sustained real damage. Let's talk more about customizing your path and the importance of starting strong.

Alejandro

Alejandro entered the university from a public high school in the same city. He was very interested in a career in medicine and had participated in a health careers program at his high school. As the first child in his family to attend college, he sought mentorship and guidance for his journey right away. For his first meeting with me, he brought in the premed track handout that the pre-health advising office had given him. According to the schedule, he needed to take Biology I with a lab and General Chemistry I with a lab his first semester, then Biology II and General Chemistry II with labs his second semester. This was nine science credits the first semester and eight science credits the second. Twelve credits is full-time. Did it make sense for Alejandro to take these courses right away when he had liberal arts, history, and writing requirements? What was he interested in studying as he adjusted to college? We talked about his science background and his high school courses. He did not have any lab classes in high school because his school did not have a science lab.

Alejandro and I created a class schedule that included an Introduction to Lab Techniques his first semester and an Introduction to General Chemistry his second semester. The rest of the courses were in writing, history, behavioral science, and recreation. Through the introductory classes he became familiar with resources in the College of Arts and Sciences and the pace of science classes in college. He did well and was able to build confidence in his ability to step up to a more rigorous schedule his second year. When it was time for him to take labs in biology, chemistry, organic chemistry, biochemistry, and physics, Alejandro was more comfortable in his surroundings, and by his third lab he served as a peer instructor. Alejandro graduated with his degree in five years— which, by the way, is the average time it takes a student in the United States to complete a bachelor's degree.[2] His grades were not a perfect 4.0, but he was well prepared and confident when he started medical school. He did not have to explain any massive blemishes on his record.

Customize Your Path

Map out a path that makes sense for *you*. Do not pressure yourself to finish or "stay on track" if that track is not your own. At most colleges these days, premed is one of the most popular major declarations for incoming first years. Thousands of students begin the journey intending on medicine as a career, but only a fraction of those remain premed at college graduation. So what goes wrong? Let's start with a little history lesson.

In 1910 a man named Abraham Flexner was hired by the American Medical Association (AMA) and the Carnegie Foundation to study medical education in the United States.[3] Before Flexner there were all types of doctors (e.g., apothecaries, bonesetters, botanists) and many pathways for training. Anyone could hang a sign up that said "doctor" and how they trained was not regulated or verified. Nothing was standardized, and although there were legitimate doctors then, there were also many bogus practitioners. The AMA was eager to standardize medicine so that the term "doctor" was consistently associated with someone who had undergone a standard training pathway. So Flexner declared in his report that a year of specific university courses should be required for entry to medical school. This began the standardization process for allopathic medicine. These course recommendations have largely gone unaltered since then.

Fast-forward to modern times where the Medical College Admissions Test (MCAT)[4] is a required element of the application. When testing was done with paper and pencil, it was only offered twice a year—April or August. Thousands of tests had to be securely collected and scanned, so it took at least eight weeks before scores were released. Applicants who took the August test were at a big disadvantage because their scores came out in October (late in the application cycle). So colleges aimed to have their students prepare for the exam in April. Back in 2000, most students applied right out of college, meaning they started during their third year of undergrad with applications and matriculated to medical school after graduating the following spring. Why does this matter?

Many university premed course tracks will set you up to finish *all* your premed courses by the first semester of your third year, despite it being unnecessary now. Even though the sequencing of the MCAT has changed, some premed course tracks have not. That's roughly five semesters to complete one year of biology, one year of general chemistry, one year of organic chemistry, one year of physics, plus biochemistry, genetics, and any other classes that schools may require. (The requirements may not be exactly the same for every medical school.) That is a formidable list of tough courses to tackle in a short period of time. The good news is that you do not have to accept a "one size fits all" format. Think about it. One size does not fit all. If we gave everyone a pair of boots that are women's size 8 and asked them to run a mile, how many people would be out of luck and unable to even make forward progress?

Please believe me when I say that you can take charge of your classes and construct a schedule that is ideal for you. Speak with your academic or prehealth adviser and ask for options. Be an advocate for yourself and your path. There are many wonderful advisers who will work with you to customize your pathway, even though it may extend your undergraduate time. Many students worry about the cost of taking another semester or two, but I promise this option is cheaper and more certain than a postbaccalaureate program down the road. (It is important to note that not all postbaccalaureate options have full financial aid and getting into programs can be competitive.)

You can also use summers strategically to plan your schedule so that your course load stays manageable. If you consider summers, you have nine semesters for classes even without a gap year (year one fall/spring/summer, year two fall/spring/summer, year three fall/spring/summer). Taking a different sequence of classes is not to say that you avoid challenges, but you should assess your earlier experience and preparations to set yourself up for success. Think of it as a runway: How much distance do you need to take off and soar to 30,000 feet?

The MCAT has been computer-based since 2005. It is offered more than twenty times a year between January and September.[5] Scores are typically released in thirty days or less. This means you do not have to take the test during your third year. You have the flexibility to complete an additional semester of courses and take it during the summer before your fourth year. If you do not plan to apply while you're working on your undergraduate degree, you have even more flexibility in deciding when you complete your courses and take the MCAT.

Nearly half of the applicants to medicine do not apply during their third year and plan to take a gap year. Many students take more than a year between graduating and applying. Students these days are beautifully curious and approach their preparation differently than in generations past. Today I see equal emphasis on the journey and the destination.

The MCAT typically has a three-year shelf life at most schools. If you plan to take time off, consider that your score should not be more than three years old when you apply. (Also be sure to check if there is an expiration on your premed course work. Some schools have a shelf life for courses as well, although that is less common.) Some students plan to apply to medical school, secure a seat, and then defer for a year to finish up other activities. While this may be a reasonable plan if you think your MCAT is going to expire, be aware that deferment requests are granted by schools on a case-by-case basis. Most of the time if there are reasonable justifications schools allow them, but they are not guaranteed. It's better to plan your test window effectively up front.

ASSESS YOUR SCIENCE BACKGROUND

So now that we have that out of the way let's talk about getting off to a strong start. Step 1: Assess your science background. Remember that "one size fits all" premed course track? Well, we need to put that in the recycle bin. You have the power to customize your journey, and you need to use it! First, take this simple quiz (see table 1.1).

If you scored a 15, you may consider taking one of your premedical courses the first semester/quarter of your first year of college, but it's not necessary. This advice may be controversial to some. You don't have to follow it, but it is honestly what I would recommend if you were my kid. Do not take any science courses during your first semester of your first year. I repeat: Do not take any of your premedical science courses out of the gate. Why would I give this advice? It takes a while to adjust to college. No matter who you are, this life adjustment is a big deal.

TABLE 1.1. Science Background Assessment

1	I took basic chemistry in high school	yes	no
2	I took advanced chemistry in high school	yes	no
3	I took basic biology in high school	yes	no
4	I took advanced biology in high school	yes	no
5	I took general physics in high school	yes	no
6	I took advanced physics in high school	yes	no
7	I took statistics in high school	yes	no
8	I took calculus in high school	yes	no
9	I took genetics in high school	yes	no
10	I earned at least a B+ in all my high school science classes	yes	no
11	My high school had a state-of-the-art lab	yes	no
12	I am familiar with basic lab equipment	yes	no
13	I am familiar with basic lab techniques	yes	no
14	I have lived on a college campus for at least 2 weeks before	yes	no
15	I have lived away from home for at least 4 weeks before	yes	no
	TOTAL yes answers:		

College Success

In my experience, succeeding in college is actually not primarily about intellectual capability. (I have a PhD and even at that level it's the same story!) Brilliance only gets you so far. Succeeding in college is about life skills, navigation, and executive function first. Learning to navigate the college environment takes time. Building skills to manage your performance in the college classroom also takes time. Developing a skill set to manage your academic performance and access the resources you need takes time. Relationships, life stress, and being away from home for the first time are all things that can really affect your performance. Consider an example.

Ari

Ari participated in a science scholars program in high school. Ari had always performed well in classes, graduated as valedictorian, then declared premed and registered for general biology and general chemistry the first semester. Ari joined several campus organizations and enthusiastically became involved in GlobeMed during freshman year, but struggled to balance academic demands with social engagements. Ari's performance started to slip after cramming to pull off Bs in classes. During first finals week in the fall semester, Ari's roommate became suicidal and Ari spent the week distracted and concerned. They did not know how to reach out for help and tried to handle the situation alone. The night before the biology final, Ari was in the emergency room with the roommate who had attempted suicide. Ari straggled in to take the final exam, unprepared and exhausted, and received a D in biology and a C in chemistry.

These grades did not reflect Ari's capacity for science or previous preparation for college science from high school. But the social factors of adjusting to college greatly affected this student's performance. Discouraged and ashamed of the poor grades, Ari did not talk to any friends or mentors about what happened. Feeling like a failure in pursuing medicine, Ari changed to sociology as a major and thrived academically from that point forward. When we met, Ari was 23 and seeking postbaccalaureate programs to get back on the path to becoming a doctor. Ari began the journey at that point, a confident, resolute, and mature student. Today Ari is happily practicing medicine. But for every positive outcome, there are countless stories of students who never circled back to their dream.

Getting off to a solid start is important for building self-efficacy in college, and there are other reasons to approach your premed coursework carefully. You will need letters of recommendation from professors who have taught you in the classroom. Many schools require letters from science professors. Getting to know professors requires maturity and engagement during class. During your first and second years you are less likely to have the skills to impress your professors. Building relationships with professors might mean going to office hours or supplemental instruction. It might mean joining a research project or volunteering as a teaching assistant or tutor. Becoming a seasoned student takes time. Grades typically improve over the course of college, so your performance is likely to be better the longer you have been in college. You will also be studying for the MCAT toward the latter half of your college career, so why front load all your science courses? It will be better to have the MCAT material fresh in your mind from your courses.

Choosing a Major

Before we leave this topic I have one more important piece of advice. You can major in anything you want. You do not have to be a science major to prepare for medicine. Advisers may encourage you to major in science or assume you wish to major in science because it is very efficient for the courses you will be required to take. This means that the requirements to complete the major and the premed requirements overlap nicely. But the best and most experienced advisers will guide you to seek a major that reflects your strengths and interests. Major in something about which you are passionate, curious, and excited. Choose more than one major if you wish! You will have more fun and likely perform better in college if you study something that you love learning on a deep level. You will still have to take the required array of premed courses, but you can diversify your undergraduate education any way you'd like. You will need to work with your adviser to ensure that you plan carefully, and you may need to use some of your major's elective options for science, but it is feasible. One class we admitted in 2017 at the Stritch School of Medicine had over fifty majors represented and it was almost an even split between science and nonscience majors.

2

Advice for First-Generation Students

I am a first-generation college graduate and professional. What I have learned working with students over the years is that everyone's journey is unique. I will talk about common pitfalls and also highlight unique strengths that can make education pioneers thrive and shine. Let's consider the stories of two first-generation students.

Haley

Haley grew up in a very unstable home. She attended fifteen schools between kindergarten and high school graduation. There were times during her childhood that her family was homeless and she lived in temporary housing and shelters. Her parents divorced and each subsequently remarried and divorced. She had three half siblings on her mom's side, two half siblings on her dad's side, and two step siblings. She began working when she turned fourteen to help support her family. She frequently gave money to family members for bills, food, drugs, alcohol, or cigarettes. Haley's family had limited capacity to teach her how to navigate the world of higher education, and they did not know how to support her college journey. They lived day to day and thought only of survival. In the home, there was a high degree of ambiguity and dysfunction in daily life. Haley grew up without routine, stability, or consistency.

When I met Haley, she was supporting her mother and working full-time while also attending college full-time. Haley's mother was not working because she "preferred to only work part-time." Haley's family was, in a word, toxic. They constantly destabilized her efforts to pursue her goals. They manipulated her into putting her car up for a title loan at 190 percent interest. They used her identity to open accounts and default on bills. She found out the hard way that her credit was a mess through no fault of her own. Haley loved her family and felt guilty every time she did not respond to their pleas for money or favors. She was aware of the drama that her family constantly inflicted, yet she struggled to distance herself from them. She did not have the skills to say no to them. She knew she wanted a different life, but she didn't quite know how to get there.

Mitch

Mitch was also a first-generation student. His father owned a plumbing company and his mother was disabled. Mitch's family had stable financial resources because of his father's business. Growing up, he lived in a suburb and attended average-quality public schools. Mitch's parents had not attended college, but they were supportive, cohesive, and stable. He lived in the same house his entire childhood. He had three younger sisters, with whom he was very close, and together they cared for their mother. He learned his father's trade growing up and began helping on various jobs when he was ten. During college he spent summers working with his father on construction and plumbing jobs. Mitch lacked knowledge to navigate the higher education system, but he had learned effective systems navigation in business and industry from his family. He had a strong, stable base from which to launch.

I want to point out that there is great diversity in first-generation students. Poverty comes in many forms, and material poverty is just one of them. There are families in higher socioeconomic strata with the same toxic emotional dynamic of Haley's, yet those students are less vulnerable because the financial hardship is not added to their struggles. Mitch and Haley will have very different learning curves coming to college and pursuing medicine. The challenges they will face will require different approaches and resources in order to overcome. Haley will need to learn new interpersonal boundaries with her family and new life skills such as budgeting and living independently. She may need counseling to cope with the trauma of her unstable childhood. Mitch and Haley will need to learn the ins and outs of college life and how to navigate the academic system, but from vastly different starting points.

What makes being a trailblazer so difficult is that you don't know what you don't know. You must rely on others to teach you new customs, norms, and habits. You must rely on mentors to light the path and show you how to navigate new environments and challenges. Being open to feedback is a key component of success. In my personal journey, I have been fortunate to have mentors and supervisors who cared enough to give me honest feedback about my performance, behavior, and approach. I sought mentors through my classes, jobs, and community. I had supervisors teach me how to conduct myself in meetings. When I wore shorts on casual Friday, my mentor let me know that it was not appropriate for our office. If you want to be a trailblazer, your ability to listen and adapt is key.

Boundaries

Let's start with one of the hardest areas for students who have experienced material and emotional poverty in their families of origin: boundaries. Cooperation and collaboration are effective survival strategies in resource scarce environments. If I am short on rent one month and you loan me money, you likely do so knowing that next time you're short on cash, I will return the favor. The problem with this model is that no one is planning to get to a stable place. By always returning a favor, you constantly obligate yourself to the cycle. Boundaries are hard. Saying no is difficult, especially when you feel you are letting someone down or not meeting their expectations. The truth is that college is hard enough just to get yourself through, and you will make it harder on yourself if you are rescuing others at the same time. Now, let's return to our example.

Haley II

Haley was living on her own for the first time at the age of 23. She had a small one-bedroom apartment and her family became aware of her situation. Soon the requests started coming in for family members to move in. She had a brother living in his car, a mother living in a shelter, and another brother who needed housing and supervision in order to be released from jail on probation. Haley was tortured to say no, but she knew that working full-time and tackling her difficult science courses required her to have a sanctuary at home. Since getting her own place she realized how important it was to live in a neat and clean environment where she had control. She no longer felt anxious at home. She slept peacefully for the first time in her life. Haley knew she could not invite the drama that would distract her and demand so much of her time and emotional energy. She considered allowing her brother to shower at her place, but she knew that it would easily lead to him sleeping there and that she would not be able to kick him out if that happened. She was firm and kept her sights on her long-term goals. She reminded herself constantly that she had to put herself and her goals first, and that was unfamiliar and uncomfortable for Haley. While most kids grow up putting their own goals first, sometimes even too much, Haley had conditioned herself to say yes, *even at her own expense*. She reviewed her list of long-term goals daily. She reinforced to herself that she could help her family in more substantial ways if she finished school and persevered to a brighter future in medicine.

Mitch II

Mitch arrived on campus motivated and well prepared. He eased himself into classes by only taking general education requirements his first year. Mitch attended all his orientation meetings and new student sessions. He took advantage of the resources on campus, especially the writing center. Even if he thought he already knew something, he went anyway; he took nothing for granted. He joined a service club his freshman year and met lifelong friends who shared his passion for community. Many of his friends were also first generation, and some had attended elite private schools on scholarships. Mitch also had friends with parents who had attended college and gone on to graduate school or professional careers. Through his peer friendships Mitch learned how to navigate college. He had a trusted group of friends who were connected to networks that could answer questions, provide advice, and offer social support. He learned to develop relationships with his professors and mentors, earning a position in a lab in his fourth year. He applied to be a mentor through the newly established First Gen office and enjoyed helping first-year students adjust to college.

Advice on Advice: Consider the Source

We live in an information-saturated world. There are many sources of advice out there and a college campus is no different. When you are a first-gen student, many people may reach out to mentor you and offer advice. You may also be accustomed to having mentors and family from home giving you advice. As you begin to navigate this journey you will need to be savvy in determining the source of your advice. A lawyer and a doctor are both considered smart people. But you would not want legal advice from a doctor or a lawyer to perform your surgery. When you are coming from a background where many in your personal network may not have gone to school, you may be less accustomed to distinguishing who is qualified to give you advice and for what.

When my twins were born, I knew I needed support. I was working full-time and working on my doctorate. I had no family living nearby and was new to Chicago. I heard about a local club for parents of multiples, so I joined. I went to the meet-ups and enjoyed getting to know fellow parents of twins and triplets. We had sessions on developmental issues, potty training, feeding, and discipline. However, sometimes when I sought advice it was not very applicable. I asked what the best double stroller was. Everyone recommended a stroller that cost over $1,400. I was driving a 1997 Nissan Sentra at the time that I knew wasn't worth that much, so I could not afford an expensive stroller. Other women recommended night nannies, "So you can get good sleep." There was a baby sleep consultant that some women highly recommended. Some of the advice given and resources recommended did not apply to me or my situation.

Here are the takeaways: 1) consider the source, 2) don't get discouraged, and 3) keep seeking. All of my fellow club members and parents of multiples were well meaning and kind. They gave the advice they knew based on their personal experiences. (That's basically the definition of advice, right?) It was not meant to disenfranchise me or make me feel left out. It just happened not to apply to my situation. I did not let their advice discourage me, I simply had to keep seeking advice until I felt I received guidance that was feasible to my situation. I enjoyed the meet-ups and friendships with my fellow club members, but when it came to advice, I learned to be selective. Eventually you will develop the ability to distinguish good advice.

Emilia

Emilia was awarded a very prestigious scholarship to attend an East Coast school. She grew up in California, the youngest daughter in an immigrant family. One of Emilia's older brothers had gone to community college near home, but she was the first to leave home for college. Her family was proud of her, but they did not want her to go away for school. They wanted her to attend a school nearby as her brother had done. Emilia really wanted to go away; she struggled with the decision but felt in her gut that it was the best thing for her and her future goals.

Adjusting to college was difficult for Emilia. The environment was new, the weather was cold, and she did not have friends or family nearby. She was very homesick during her first semester and called home nearly every day. Her family would sympathize with her and listen to her fears and woes. Their advice to her each time they heard her strife was, "Come home." After a tough semester, Emilia withdrew, moved home, and gave up her scholarship.

Rather than focus her energy on settling into her new environment, Emilia continued to anchor toward home. In order to move forward, she needed to build a support network and wade through the initial hard phase of adjusting to school. She needed to talk to people who had successfully navigated the challenges she was facing: an expert on adjusting to school away from home, or perhaps another first-generation student. Her family loved her deeply, but they had no expertise to provide advice on her challenges adjusting to college. Their advice was well intentioned, but it was not what Emilia needed to achieve the goals that she had set for herself when she made the choice to attend school on the East Coast.

Questions for Advice Seekers

If you are a savvy resource seeker, you will develop skills to discern whether to accept advice. Ask yourself these questions when seeking advice.

- Is this person an expert on the subject about which I am asking? (Assess expertise based on tangible evidence, reputation, and endorsements from others within the same field.)
- Does this person have experience with my issue? (Directly ask them if they have experience with your issue or situation.)
- Is this person invested in my success? (Do they care if I succeed or fail? Are they personally invested in me? How well do they know me?)
- Can I corroborate their advice with that of another invested expert?
- Does this expert share or understand aspects of my background and identity that may relate to my challenge?

I am not saying that Emilia should not have called home. What I am saying is that Emilia should have been clear and intentional about seeking support for her goals. Family members can be a great source of validation and emotional support, but they may not be the right source of advice if you are struggling with biochemistry or a professor who is unfair. Before you seek advice, step back and identify your problem. Then examine the advisers and resources available to you and select the right expert.

Work with Your Prehealth Adviser

If you are fortunate to attend a university with a prehealth adviser, you should begin to build a relationship with the adviser as soon as possible. Whether you are automatically assigned one or your school requires you to register with the office, you should get started right away. Many first-generation students do not realize the importance of meeting with career counselors and advisers early in their college years. I met with an adviser my first year because it was required in order to register for classes. I did not seek help again until my final semester, which is when I learned I had to take two math classes in order to graduate. Oops. I worked during school and was very busy; I did not approach college with a career mindset because I did not know I was supposed to. My finish line was my bachelor's degree because I did not realize there was a whole educational world beyond that.

Not all schools have prehealth advising services and savvy mentors to help guide premedical students. Prehealth advising structures can vary from school to school; your options may be a single faculty member that guides students informally to an extensive career development program run by many staff members and faculty. Find out what your school offers. Ask if there is a prehealth committee process that you may need to engage in order to receive a prehealth committee letter. If there is a committee process it will likely help you become a stronger applicant.

PREHEALTH COMMITTEES

A prehealth committee is comprised of a group of faculty members and experts that evaluate a cohort of students applying to graduate or professional programs. The committee usually has a program where applicants meet certain requirements that align with the application process, such as personal statements describing experiences and letters of recommendation. There may be mock interviews, application workshops, or other resources associated with the committee process. Some committees rank and categorize their students, others simply offer an evaluative summary of the preparation areas and main strengths of an applicant. If your school has such a committee, it's a good idea to follow that process. However, if you do not go through the committee process it does not mean you cannot apply.

The positives of prehealth committees are many, but there can be a downside. Some committees may have academic minimums that students must meet to qualify for a committee evaluation and letter. As an admissions dean I wholeheartedly disagree with this practice. I would like applicants to apply so that my faculty committee can evaluate them; I do not appreciate the prehealth committees applying cutoffs that my faculty may not have applied in the first place. Committees may also have deadlines that do not accommodate the lives of students and are therefore too rigid for students to meet. For example, if a student is not sure whether they will be applying in May and they miss the committee deadline, they are faced with applying without a committee letter or waiting a year. There may be other contingencies affecting whether or not a student can use their school's prehealth committee.

Rest assured, you cannot be restricted from applying to medical school by your university. Medical schools usually do not disqualify applicants without committee letters, since some schools do not have them. You do not have to go through the committee process, since you are free to get letters of recommendation using the American Medical College Application Service (AMCAS) portal[1] or another letter service for advisers or other letter authors. If you choose not to use premed advising or committee services at your school, you may be asked the reason why later on in the process (perhaps in an interview), particularly if the school is well known for having strong, active advising. If you have a reasonable response you will not be penalized. Most committees are going to evaluate you based on YOU, not your school.

Here is another important fact: The statistics provided by your premed advising office are only for students who have worked with their office and agreed to disclose their information. An adviser at the undergraduate level has no idea that you are applying unless you tell them. They are not allowed to get information from medical schools about your status unless you explicitly agree to share it. Hopefully you are able to rely on wonderful advisers for the journey, but if not, don't be discouraged.

THE ROLE OF THE ADVISER

Ask what information and resources the prehealth advising office has for you. Advisers can advocate for you and help you customize your path. They usually know insider information about professors, courses, and the pathway at your institution. They know about sequencing of classes and important deadlines. Maybe you are planning to start your physics sequence in the spring—your adviser will be able to tell you that the sequence only starts in the fall. There are countless details like this that advisers can help you with that will ultimately make your journey better. Advisers also have good information about where students from your school have gone to medical school and which medical schools may give you the most consideration. They can help you avoid pitfalls and open doors of opportunity for you. They may have workshops, shadowing programs, community referrals, and other resources to help in your exploration and preparation.

As an admissions dean, I value my relationships with advisers. Advisers, by and large, are passionate and committed to your success. They are thrilled when their students achieve their goals. On many instances I have called an adviser to follow up about a candidate. My committee may strongly support that individual but we have some lingering questions or concerns. It is a tremendous resource to be able to speak with someone the applicant has authorized to represent them in order to alleviate a concern. The more the adviser knows you, the better able they are to advocate for you.

Marnie

Marnie was a candidate in our admissions process. I was preparing her file for committee and noticed comments on the interview reports about her interpersonal demeanor. Both interviewers had noted that Marnie was very shy and may lack self-confidence. Although the interview reports were fair, they expressed concerns about how the candidate would perform in group settings or how she would go about establishing rapport with patients. I pulled the adviser letter and called Marnie's adviser. She was on vacation and her assistant agreed to forward a message for me.

The fact that the very next day the adviser called me while on vacation illustrates just how invested many advisers are in their students' successes. Marnie's adviser provided more detail about Marnie's personality and people skills. She gave specific examples of personal interactions she had observed over Marnie's undergraduate years. I shared these remarks with the committee at the next meeting and Marnie received an offer of admission. I cannot stress enough how much you should work to use the resources that your prehealth office provides, including building a relationship with your adviser.

You should also know I do not penalize applicants who attend schools where there are no prehealth advisers. I completely understand that applicants do the best with what they have; not having an adviser is beyond your control. If your school lacks a prehealth adviser, do your best to get to know professors so that you can have strong individual letters when you apply. At most schools you will not be penalized for not having a premed committee letter. However, for students who attend schools where we know there is a strong, active adviser, we might wonder why that student has chosen to apply outside the advising structure. If this is you, you may aid your candidacy if you explain in your supplemental why you chose not to seek a committee letter or why you chose not to work with your premed adviser.

Cautions about Advisers

For all the positive stories about advisers, unfortunately there are also negative ones. It may seem contradictory that I just said to work closely with your adviser and now I am going to caution you. But the reality is that not all advisers are created equal. Not all universities provide the resources necessary to support premedical students with strong advising. Sometimes there is a lack of knowledge, investment, or both on the part of those charged with supporting premed students. This is why you must be a savvy advice seeker.

Aaron

Aaron went to see his premed adviser during his second year. He had a 2.92 grade point average after first year and was feeling confident about his science courses that semester, despite earning one C. He was excited to talk about his path and wanted advice on how else to prepare. The adviser looked at his grades and told Aaron that he would never get into medical school because his grades were already out of range for medicine and that he should change his major and choose something else. Thankfully, Aaron did not listen to this adviser. Although the person was a subject expert appointed by the school, he was not invested in Aaron personally and did not take the time to get to know Aaron.

You will be happy to know that Aaron went on to perform well in college and continued his premed path. He found other mentors and faculty champions who were invested in his success. When he applied he tactfully explained that he had faced some discouragement from well-meaning advisers at his school. At the end of the process he had multiple offers for medical school. He is now a prestigious subspecialist in his field.

You are the keeper of your dreams. Remember, these people are largely not ill-intentioned. The best advisers help you with the *how* of achieving your goals. The best advisers get to know you personally before collaboratively helping you make decisions about your future. It should not be the business of advisers to dictate what they think you can or cannot do. Advisers should provide feedback about your plans and help you execute them. If an adviser is cautioning you, they probably have your best interest in mind. You should step back and assess the situation together with your adviser to be sure you both fully understand all parameters and details of the choices at hand.

There have been many times I have had difficult advising appointments giving feedback that I know the student did not want to hear. I always do my best to emphasize my support for their long-term goals, and my willingness to tell the truth is a demonstration that I take their goals seriously. I know that advisers can get a bad rap for telling the truth, and ironically it's often the best advisers that will indeed be truthful with you. Make sure that if you choose not to work with an adviser it is because you have had a direct, personal experience. Do not write someone off based on rumors or another person's story.

If someone is discouraging you, step back and assess their place in your life. Your inclination to accept a path-change from an adviser should be highly related to your personal relationship with them and your confidence that they will be continually invested in you even after you make that choice. In other words, only consider drastic advice from people that you know really love and care about you. Give your prehealth adviser a chance and work to get to know them. Don't give up or let someone discourage your dreams.

Successful Students Access Resources

College campuses are filled with marvelous resources to help students succeed. When I discovered that there were reference librarians who could help me find books and journal articles for the papers I was assigned to write, my college life got a whole lot easier. As a first-generation student you may not know what resources are out there, so the first step is to find out. Is there a tutoring center? A writing center? A counseling center? A fitness center? Make sure you know what your school provides so that you can take advantage of all these resources. Your tuition and fees are paying for them. They are there because students need them and use them. Do not fall into the trap of believing that you are somehow less if you use them.

I like to tell students that not using your campus resources is like having a closet full of new clothes and not wearing them. You have already paid for these aspects of college life. Why would you not use them? Your physical, social, emotional, and spiritual health are all critical to your academic success. Take care of yourself and get the help you need when you need it. If there are aspects of your personal development—whether academic, social, or spiritual—that need work, a college campus is a great place to plug into resources and improve.

3
Advice for Minoritized Students

The history of allopathic medicine in the United States explains a great deal about the landscape of the profession today. If you would like to know more, I recommend you read up on Abraham Flexner,[1] the American Medical Association's council on medical education, and the Carnegie Foundation. (I did my dissertation[2] on allopathic medicine, and in the second chapter give a thorough summary of the pre- and post-Flexner era.) Let me give you the short version here. Medicine has a long history of exclusionary practices that favored powerful groups: White, male, heterosexual, upper class, urban. Visit any medical school that has been around for fifty years or more and the walls will tell you what I mean. You can look through the archives of the *Journal of the American Medical Association* and find articles written in the late 1800s seeking to make medicine more exclusive and elite.[3] If you don't fit the profile of the founders of allopathic medicine, you may find yourself underrepresented in various contexts of your journey and minoritized by the institutions and structures that have created the system we have today. While medicine now recognizes the value of inclusion and is striving to recruit and train a diverse physician workforce, the vestiges of bias remain—both blatant and latent. Many systems and institutional climates are not designed with inclusion in mind.

What do I mean by minoritized? Why don't I just say "minority" or "underrepresented minority"? I believe that our identities are fluid and intersectional. There are spaces we inhabit where we feel we belong and spaces we enter where we feel on the outside. This is not only a function of who we are, but also a consequence of the context we inhabit. There are settings where I feel my identity as a woman is quite salient, like when I am coaching my daughter's basketball team in a league of sixteen teams and I am the only head coach who is a woman. It is not that my identity as a female makes me a minority, it's that the situation potentially places me on the margins or under more scrutiny than other coaches. In that setting I am acutely aware of my gender identity and gender expression.

We know that there are many groups historically underrepresented in medicine. If you have grown up not seeing yourself reflected in medicine and healthcare settings, we need you. Your background, experiences, perspectives, and talents are needed to build a physician workforce that will meet the needs of all patients. I am telling you this from my very core with all the passion I can muster. I have dedicated my life to ensuring diversity and opportunity in medicine. If medicine is your dream, you owe it to your future patients to work hard and persevere. You are needed. Medicine belongs to you, too.

Common Pitfalls

I am going to address some common pitfalls I have seen over the years related to minoritization. I would like for you to be immune (as much as possible) from some of these distractions and assaults on your goals. Be resilient and forewarned in the face of some of these challenges.

FIRST TIP: STUPID AND HAVEN'T LEARNED IT YET ARE NOT THE SAME THING

I traveled to Washington, D.C., for one of my very first professional conferences when I was in my early twenties. I had not traveled much in my life, let alone solo. (I took my first airline flight when I was seventeen and was thirty-six years old when I got my passport.) I grew up in the suburbs where parents taxied their children from place to place until their children could drive. I had never hailed a cab or rode a city bus, a train, or subway. I spoke with a few colleagues who were flying in from other schools about the trip. They told me to take the D.C. Metro from the airport to the hotel because it was very easy. "Just follow the signs," they said. So I got off the plane and followed the airport signs to the Metro. I stood in the boarding area, looking at several transit maps for various train lines, and realized I had no idea whatsoever how to ride the train. In that moment I was completely overwhelmed. Afraid I would end up somewhere else (in New Jersey!), I bailed on my plan to take the train and made my way back to the taxi stand instead.

Did I fail at taking the train? Yes, I did. But was it because I was stupid? No. Did I find a way to get where I was going? Yes. Not knowing how to do something is not the same thing as being stupid. Sometimes when we are in new environments we allow these experiences to be internalized and make us feel inadequate or "less than." Do not fall into this thinking error. What makes a person stupid or smart has more to do with the knowledge they have acquired in the past and their current ability to learn. As you approach your classes and experiences, recognize that you are learning. Give yourself space to learn and permission to not be perfect the first time you do something. Rather than say that you are not good at something, say you are learning instead. "I'm not good at networking" should be "I'm learning how to network," or "I am improving my networking skills." These are more accurate statements than framing your abilities as finite and inflexible.

Realize that the experiences you have and the knowledge from those experiences is valuable. It may not directly apply to the context you are in during a college course or a professional meeting, but that does not mean it is not valuable. Especially in medicine, when one of your primary skills is relating to patients, your experiences will be invaluable moving forward.

Danesh

Danesh was interviewing a patient with his care team of fellow third year medical students. The patient interview was going well and the team was gathering relevant information. Danesh asked the patient about his drinking habits. The patient responded that he drinks "a fifth of whiskey a day, sometimes more." Everyone on Danesh's team wrote copious notes and later presented to the attending physician about what they had learned, their differential diagnoses, and plans of care. Danesh's patient presentation included relevant information about the patient's heavy drinking and how it related to his current condition and subsequent care plan. His classmates did not include information related to the patient's drinking. Later, when the team was finished with the consultation, Danesh asked his classmates why they did not think the drinking was a relevant detail. They said they did not know what a fifth was. Danesh was astounded. He was happy to inform them that it was 750 milliliters and about sixteen shots. His classmates felt silly that they had left out such a drastic aspect of the patient's history. Danesh's experiences growing up in the central valley of California had yielded different knowledge than his peers. He had worked at a convenience store in his community during high school.

There will be times when you are on the "know" side and the "don't know" side of the coin throughout your journey. Do not allow the times you do not know something to take away your confidence. You are where you are because of your ability to learn and grow, not because you showed up already knowing everything. The environment you are in may not recognize all you have to offer, but it will be valuable down the road. In the meantime, keep learning and approaching new experiences with confidence and openness. You will find that your bandwidth for relating to people increases as you learn and grow.

SECOND TIP: UNDERSTAND STEREOTYPE THREAT

If you have not heard of stereotype threat (ST), you need to know about it. Claude Steele's book *Whistling Vivaldi*[4] provides a very detailed summary of the research on ST and also what is known about combating it. The basics are this: When you are in an identity-salient situation where you have the potential to confirm a negative stereotype about yourself, it can affect your performance without your consciously realizing it. Stereotype threat arises out of a situation where your identity as it relates to your task becomes relevant and thus distracts your mind from higher-order processing. Here is an example of how it works.

Let's say we take a group of older adults (age 65+) and give them a memory test using an online game. The first time we give them the test we tell them that we are testing a new game to see how well it works. We record their scores. Now we are going to test them again, only this time when we ask them to do the online memory game we tell them that we are doing research on dementia. This introduces a stereotype threat that people who are aging have dementia or diminished mental capacity around memory. The second set of scores is lower than the first. This is ST's effect on performance.

Stereotype threat is universal across all populations. It depends on the situation, but it can affect both physical and mental tasks. Studies have been done on everything from athletes and mini-golf,[5] White men and jumping,[6] to IQ tests.[7] The results continually show performance decrements when under ST. The task has to be difficult and the people doing it have to care about the task. The more you care about the task, the greater the effect on performance can be. You can see how this might be a pitfall for minoritized students in college. Well, it turns out that just being aware of it can help, so you have completed your first intervention.

To protect yourself against ST you have to be in charge of your mind. Affirmations and positive self-talk are important. You must think of all the ways that you are similar to those around you, rather than different. In a class where you feel you are alone in your identity, try to find similarities. Everyone is a science major, everyone is premed, everyone is challenged by the work.

Recognize that you are only seeing a partial version of reality. Everyone on campus is accessing resources in order to be successful. Period. Do not fall into the trap of thinking that you are studying your tail off while everyone else is so magically brilliant that they are pulling A grades without studying. I don't care what their Instagram says; they are studying! And do not compare yourself to others, because you usually won't have all the information for an accurate comparison.

Paula

Paula got an 81 percent on her first exam in medical school and was pretty bummed that she did not do better. She understood the material but was feeling down about her score. As we chatted in the office some of her peers came by. They started talking about the exam as well. Paula learned that some of her classmates had access to old notes through someone's sibling who was in the class above them. She had been comparing her scores to the scores of students who had an advantage. All of a sudden she realized her 81 percent was pretty damn good, since she earned it without the benefit of knowing what was on the test beforehand. She stayed focused on her learning first, and let her performance be what it may. She studied to master material, not to get high grades or honors. When it came time to take the USMLE Step 1 (United States Medical Licensing Examination), Paula sat with confidence and scored in the 95th percentile. Had she allowed a false comparison to throw her off her game, she might not have performed to her potential.

THIRD TIP: SELF-CARE AND RESILIENCE AT AN HWCU

Many of you are likely familiar with what it feels like to attend a Historically White College or University (HWCU). These institutions were not designed with a diverse population of students in mind. Structurally and traditionally, many of these schools have artifacts of White supremacy that are extremely hard to eradicate. It's like lead in the environment. We all know it's toxic, and yet lead has not been eliminated even with concerted efforts. These are micro-aggressions, micro-insults, and micro-invalidations that over time can really wear you down. From the names of buildings on campuses to the food served in the cafeteria, you are confronted each day with micro-messages that you do not belong. It can be hard to be resilient in the face of daily micro-assaults on your identity. You have to build resilience and attend to self-care in order to thrive. One of my students called it putting up "hater blockers." You have to be mentally prepared to encounter biases and disconnects along the way.

Albert

Albert was a third year student rotating on internal medicine. His team had just seen an HIV-positive patient who also identified as gay. As they were walking to their next patient room, he heard one of the residents use derogatory language about the patient and his partner. Albert was upset. As a Black man who is gay, he could not believe what he was hearing, and yet he struggled to know what to do because of his identity. If he confronted the senior residents, he would risk being outcast or receiving poor grades. Yet knowing their biases felt terrible. Albert felt alone and upset that he had somehow failed to stand up for his patient and his community. He came to my office to vent. Through our conversation he was able to put the experience in perspective and become aware of the resources at the school for reporting and challenging unprofessional behavior. Albert was not in a position of power, but he channeled his frustration into action. He helped create a training course to educate staff, faculty, residents, and students at his school about health disparities within the LGBTQ community. The course became a permanent offering at his school.

These situations are incredibly difficult, and they also happen all too often. There is no right way or wrong way to handle them. No one has the right to judge you for what you did or did not do in that moment. But you absolutely must process these inputs and handle them in a way that allows you not to get bogged down, distracted, angry, and depressed. Easier said than done, right?

Build your support team and make sure it includes excellent listeners. These folk are the ones with whom you can talk about anything and they will not try to convince you that your reality isn't valid. These people will believe you and authentically validate you.

These crucial listeners help you process your experiences and also help you not carry the weight of them moving forward. A support team empathizes with you and encourages you when you are down.

Support team members can be classmates, significant others, family members, mentors, or friends. My students in the past have found support in their faith-based communities, sororities, and yoga studios. Students have joined supper clubs, marathon training teams, or martial arts dojos to find positive outlets. Sometimes students prefer solo time painting, meditating, crocheting, or walking. Most schools also have counseling services available to students for free, which I highly recommend that you use.

Create a web of support outside of premed and medicine. The path to medicine is long and arduous. It helps to have a life outside of that path that is also authentic to who you are. One of my colleagues is an avid bird-watcher. She attends meetings of like-minded folk where I am certain no one talks about surgery or medicine. Outlets create balance and allow you to feel validation and connection outside of your chosen vocation. This is vital. There are so many communities in which you can be meaningfully engaged that will provide an escape and a validation outside of premed and medicine. Find one.

Attend to spiritual practices or your own rituals of self-care. If they help you cope, keep doing these things. If you cannot name at least three things you do to care for yourself, it's time to reassess your priorities and do better. I am not saying your self-care has to be an expensive spa day or a shopping habit. Self-care can be simple—like taking walks, reading library books for leisure, or routinely calling a friend. When you go through transitions, anchor yourself with your proven rituals for coping. Do not make the mistake of thinking you can be fine without implementing your previous recipe for success.

Lydia

Lydia became an emergency medical technician (EMT) before attending medical school. She loved working in her community and being a first responder. As she gained experience on a busy ambulance service, Lydia found herself emotionally taxed by some of the traumas and difficult cases she had seen. She decided that she needed a way to honor those stories without carrying them as burdens. Lydia created a pebble jar. She dedicated pebbles to patients, and the symbolic drop of the pebble into the jar was a way for her to let go. At the end of each shift, she would spend a few moments thinking of the patients she had served and their various stories, situations, and outcomes. When the jar was full, Lydia would take it to her favorite lake and leave the pebbles on the shore. This was how she learned to process some difficult experiences she had as an EMT—experiences that certainly prepared her for coping as a physician.

There are countless rituals, hobbies, and practices for self-care. Develop your own and be intentional about them. They will keep you focused and resilient amid the challenges you will face during preparation, training, and practice. While at times you may feel minoritized, you will also find wonderful allies along the way who are ready to help and support your journey.

4

Advice for Undocumented Students

As I have said before, everything I know about best practices, strategies, and advice has come from working directly with students,[1] and the advice in this chapter is no exception. While all of the advice in this book applies to undocumented students, there are some aspects of the journey that are unique to students who are undocumented and that need to be addressed. I have written this chapter inclusively, acknowledging that the undocumented student community is diverse and includes individuals recognized under the DACA (Deferred Action for Childhood Arrivals) program, those without DACA, in temporary statuses, and those who are otherwise experiencing uncertainty and ambiguity with regard to status. Now let's get down to the practical.

Undocumented with DACA

If you are undocumented with DACA and you are wondering if it is possible to become a physician, I emphatically say *yes*! I personally know of several medical school graduates who are DACA recipients and who are now practicing as physicians or resident trainees. There are articles in *Academic Medicine* acknowledging this fact and offering guidance.[2] The work authorization granted through DACA is the key to being able to complete both medical school and residency training. Residents are paid trainees, usually through hospital systems, academic medical centers, or outpatient clinics. After they match they are on-boarded by a graduate medical education office that uses hiring paperwork to verify federal employment eligibility.

Undocumented without DACA

Students without DACA face additional challenges when pursuing medicine. Medical school can be accessible if students are able to secure funding for tuition and if a school is willing to consider their application under its admissions guidelines. The American Medical College Application Service (AMCAS) has an option in the citizenship field that allows applicants to indicate a variety of statuses, but many schools may positively filter for the statuses they allow in their admissions guidelines. If you have an interim status you may need to call the school to ask about your eligibility to apply and how much consideration your application will receive. Because residency training currently requires work authorization, the pathway beyond earning the MD degree is uncertain. As this book goes to press there are no residency training options for individuals without work authorization. This means that practicing medicine (seeing patients and doing clinical work) would not be possible. This does not mean that earning an MD is not worth it. There are advocates currently working at every level to reform immigration laws in our country and to change policies that may lead to greater options. There are undocumented students without DACA currently in medical school in the United States. You are not alone.

That said, the barriers are real and it is complicated and ever-changing. My goal is always to be as honest and transparent about the path so that you have what you need to make choices and plans. You might already know the landscape of your path, but I will start at the beginning.

Application Strategy

The application strategy for undocumented students should include specific attention to the mission of the school beyond what a typical applicant might consider. As a prospective student you not only want to know that you are eligible to apply, but also whether the school has supportive structures and people there to serve as allies in changing or challenging times. Remember that if you are fortunate to earn a seat you will be a student for at least four years, and there are external factors beyond your control. Ideally there are committed individuals, transparent policies, and allies in positions of power that you can rely on if needed.

The eligibility criteria for applying can usually be found on a school's website and will include whether the school considers applications for DACA recipients or applications from undocumented students meeting other criteria, such as California's Assembly Bill (AB) 540, or the California Nonresident Tuition Exemption.[3] The Association of American Medical Colleges (AAMC) operates the Medical School Admission Requirements (MSAR) Online[4] and has information about whether a school will consider applications from DACA recipients. Note that this information published online is only for consideration of applications and does not indicate whether there are undocumented students currently enrolled or if there are institutionally sponsored financial aid options available to undocumented students. If you would like to join a community of undocumented students aspiring toward health professions, I recommend the Pre-Health Dreamers community (PHDreamers.org). Through this network you can find mentors and resources and learn where undocumented students are enrolled in medical school, dental school, and physical therapy school.

Disclosing Your Status

The AMCAS application provides an option to indicate your status in the citizenship section. There are inclusive categorical options, including DACA, Refugee, and Other, for example. You must answer this question truthfully in order to apply through AMCAS. The rules of using the application service specifically require that applicants attest to the truthfulness of their applications. Schools have the right to withdraw consideration if applicants are found to have not been truthful. You should answer truthfully for whatever your status is at the time you submit. If you have petitions or applications pending, you might choose to disclose that somewhere in the written portion of your application. If your status changes during the cycle, you can contact schools individually to update them, but AMCAS does not allow you to make changes to this aspect of your file after submission. If your status changes during the cycle and you become eligible for federal financial aid, you should inform the schools to which you have applied.

Whether or not you choose to disclose your status on the written portion of your application is entirely up to you. Some applicants feel that their motivation for medicine is intimately related to their experiences as undocumented persons and therefore choose to make this identity central in the application. Others may mention it as part of their journey but focus on another aspect that they feel is more central. There is no right or wrong here. Authenticity is key. Do understand that everything in your application is fair game for schools to ask about during interview. If you are not comfortable discussing your status openly, consider that as you put together your application. If you make it central in your writing, it is much more likely to become a topic during interview.

As is the case with all sensitive aspects of identity, applicants often ask me if it is a good strategy to be open. My answer is always the same, "Would you like to attend a school for four years that would hold this aspect of your existence or identity against you? Would you feel comfortable in an environment that did not value this part of who you are?" Think about it. You cannot be everything to all schools. Getting in at all costs may have a big downside. This journey will likely have a better ending if you represent yourself authentically so that you find a school that is the right fit in the end.

Programs and Services

Undocumented students should connect with their respective campus resources if available. Many campuses have Dream Centers—offices specifically dedicated to serving and supporting undocumented students. Undocumented students are able to register for AAMC services such as the Medical College Admission Test (MCAT), AMCAS, and the Electronic Residency Application Service (ERAS). DACA recipients are eligible for the Fee Assistance Program (FAP) if they meet the income qualifications. Undocumented students are able to submit to background checks if they have passports from their countries of origin, social security numbers issued through DACA, or other forms of official ID. Undocumented students are also able to register for licensing exams, such as the United States Medical Licensing Examination (USMLE) and those offered through the National Board of Medical Examiners (NBME). Sometimes background checks specify that students must have a social security number and/or driver's license, but usually if you let the company know that you have another form of identification they can still conduct the background check. DACA recipients have successfully completed the background check required for training at Veterans Administration health facilities. Licensure varies by state, but it is worth noting that some states, such as California, allow applications for professional licenses using individual tax identification numbers (ITINs).[5] For current information on licensure by state for undocumented professionals, I recommend contacting the National Immigrant Law Center (nilc.org).

Financial Aid

As you are well aware, undocumented students are not eligible for federal financial aid. You may be eligible for some forms of state-based aid, which can be determined on a state-by-state basis and is ever-changing. Private scholarships, private loans, grants, and educational stipends are often inclusive of undocumented students. If the criteria do not specifically address eligibility for undocumented students, contact the organization or program and ask. The progress made to date by activists and allies began with an ask.

Undocumented students have been exceptionally creative and resourceful in securing funding for school. Students have used private loans, community-based loans, grants, scholarships, crowd-sourcing, and/or creative combinations of any of these options. Be aware that private loans and some community options usually require a cosigner who is a U.S. citizen or permanent resident. Interest rates for alternative funding can also be quite high, so seek guidance from a financial aid expert to ensure you understand the terms of your loans. Ask questions and ensure you fully understand the terms before signing promissory notes.

It is ideal to have a plan for how you will fund all four years of your education when you start medical school. Sometimes situations and plans change, but it is best to begin with a long-term plan in mind so that the stressors of financing your education do not become a burden and distraction during medical school. The coursework is difficult enough without added stress about paying tuition or rent. Working during medical school is not advised, because it takes away from the critical hours needed for studying and self-care.

If you encounter funding difficulties during medical school it is possible to take a leave and stop out, but this is more common in undergrad. Stopping out is not advisable and is usually only allowed once. Most students who take a leave do so to complete research, additional degrees, or fellowships. There are opportune times to take a leave, but also times that are not ideal because of how the curriculum is delivered and the timing of licensing exams. Having supportive deans and administrators to help you navigate these unforeseen aspects is absolutely critical.

Reaching for Allies

The journeys of undocumented students are filled with stories of allies who stood up, spoke out, and were unconditionally committed to supporting students. Some students are comfortable reaching out and building support networks, and some less so. I have met many students through programs and events for undocumented students who revealed that it was the first time they had ever disclosed their status, talked openly with other undocumented students, or attended an event that was advertised for them. Being able to connect with others with similar journeys is powerful—your fellow undocumented students are some of your most powerful and knowledgeable allies. Some of the previously mentioned organizations are effective for connecting with fellow students, who in turn might know of safe and reliable allies within the ranks of administrators, deans, staff, and professors at various institutions.

Assessing Allyship

It can be risky and difficult to determine who to trust if you need help navigating systems from allies who are not themselves undocumented. Besides getting an endorsement from fellow students, try looking for signs of allyship in the physical office or social media presence of the person. What is on their office walls? What does their bio or profile say? What types of organizations do they interface with? Are there any indicators of their political leanings? You might find obvious labels, like the "Dreamers Welcome" butterfly sticker outside my door. You can also look for other social justice ally indicators that might mean someone is open to supporting you, such as evidence of their solidarity with LGBTQ persons, Black Lives Matter, and immigrants.

Accepting support from a committed ally is powerful. There are allies out there who are willing to help if you share your story and reach out. Building networks of support is critical in progressing toward your goal; no one navigates the premed journey alone, whether undocumented or not. As you reach for allies, understand that you will be educating them along the way. Even the most committed allies don't walk in your shoes and may need your truth to make course corrections. You may need to be explicit about the sensitivity of your status because not everyone will understand the complexity and vulnerability of your situation.

Jerica

Jerica came to our summer applicant boot camp and was thrilled to be there. She knew that my school was welcoming to DACA recipients and that my school had several DACA recipients currently in medical school. My school was a committed institution and had made a stand publicly to welcome DACA recipients. It was a safe space, and a school with many allies among the faculty, staff, and students. Jerica was excited to be in our program, although she was somewhat cautious because she had never publicly disclosed her status.

During the program the teaching assistants, whom I supervised, had arranged a special off-schedule session for the DACA students. They let the students know individually when the session would be held and that it was being presented by two current second year students who were DACA recipients. Because of a last-minute change in schedule, the teaching assistants announced to the entire class that the DACA session was rescheduled and asked that the DACA recipients in the summer program, including Jerica, leave lunch early to attend. This meant that Jerica's status was outed as she exited the classroom with six students.

Jerica was upset, and rightfully so. She came to my office and asked to meet with me after the session was over. I listened as she told me what had happened. She expressed that she felt unsafe, vulnerable, and that her privacy had been violated. She explained that her family is extremely private about her and her sister's status. She had never told a soul she was undocumented and essentially was forced to reveal her status to more than thirty students she had just met. She was understanding of the fact that it was not intentional, and she was professional in her feedback, but she shared fully what the experience was like for her.

I felt terrible. I apologized and accepted full responsibility for my team and our mistakes. I thanked her for trusting me and caring enough to tell me that my program had made this mistake. I explained that we had assumed our lens of the school as a safe space was everyone's lens, and that this was neither accurate nor fair to her. I committed to do better as an ally and to train my teaching assistants and staff better so that they fully understood the gravity of privacy concerns for undocumented students. I asked if there was anything I could do to make the situation right. She said that more awareness and sensitivity moving forward was what she wanted, and we both agreed to give our all to the boot camp in hopes that her application that season would be successful.

Jerica had stepped out of her comfort zone and had come to our program because she was passionate about her dream of medicine. I was the first person she confided in about her status, but I was not the last. Jerica was a top student that summer and had three offers for medical school that year. She chose to attend my school and join the community that she knew would embrace her and support her dreams. Although initially it had not gone exactly according to her plans, she trusted us enough to tell us her truth. I am grateful to this day that she judged us by our actions and visible commitment to undocumented students, and that she forgave our mistakes.

Trust but Verify

Another important aspect is to ensure that you verify what institutional leaders and student support personnel have told you. The nature of the circumstances for undocumented students often means that policies are being established for the first time or adapted on the fly, so communication gaps are possible between leaders who are otherwise well meaning and committed. It may also mean that there could be a mix of personnel who are not supportive and these personnel gaps can have negative consequences on your experience. Students calling schools to verify their eligibility to apply, for example, may get a different answer depending on the day they call and the person who picks up the phone. Sometimes there are progressive, committed leaders within institutions, but their sphere of influence may not extend to all levels of personnel. A school may have a policy and may not have informed and trained the staff and faculty. You must be savvy in how you navigate this situation.

Try to verify what one person has told you with another person within the school. Look for allies with roles directly related to supporting you and your experience as a medical student. It is a good sign if your allies are directly involved in the care and keeping of students. If the person making you promises does not supervise the personnel assigned to deliver those promises, that should be a red flag. *Always obtain information in writing.* I cannot stress this enough. Especially as it pertains to financial support, scholarships, and offers of admission—you need these agreements and offers documented in official correspondence. I have met students who acted on verbal agreements and found themselves in precarious positions because the individuals making the promises were not able to keep them. The promises were well meaning, but the individuals making them failed to go through proper institutional channels. Trust your allies, but verify agreements and promises.

Moving Forward in Uncertain Times

As this book goes to press there are pending court cases and an ever-changing landscape for undocumented students. Residency training for undocumented students without work authorization (trainees without DACA or another form of relief that provides a work permit) is uncertain. Licensure in some states is uncertain. While I cannot promise immediate results or policy changes that will guarantee smooth sailing, I can promise that I will never stop fighting for you. You should know that there are many advocates and activists working on finding solutions to ensure your access to higher education and medical education. You belong. You deserve to pursue your dreams in medicine as any student does. You bring much-needed perspectives, knowledge, and insights to medicine.

Undocumented students have taught me that pursuing your dreams amid uncertainty is the norm for them. If every step of the way is not outlined, just keep moving forward. Education is powerful and transformative. Your stories are equally powerful. As one student said to me at the very beginning, "Share your story. People may not agree, but they can never deny having heard your story. For that moment they will see your humanity and it will make a difference." I hope that we can open more avenues in the future and create pathways to medical education for undocumented students. Our communities are waiting for doctors just like you.

PART II

The Premed Journey

5
Exploration and Affirmation

Choosing a career is one of the most important decisions you will ever make. Do not skip the exploration phase of this decision. Is it wise to choose a life partner after only one date? Or after only reading about them online and watching movies about them? Probably not. A career is no different. You must carefully vet that career against your goals in life and your talents, interests, proclivities, and abilities.

Mindy

Mindy was a third year college student who came to our applicant boot camp in June, planning to apply the following month. She had strong grades and test scores and experiences in college, and her sights were firmly set on medicine. As we began writing prompts for the personal statement, Mindy struggled. She wrote draft after draft of her personal statement and each one continued to fall short in her eyes and in the eyes of the teaching assistants. She sat in my office one afternoon very distraught at her "boring writing" and the "lack of flair" in her application. She had discussed all her wonderful experiences and extrapolated her very robust resume, but her essays never answered the most important question: why she wanted to be a doctor. She provided a generic answer about solving puzzles, loving science, and always knowing that was what she wanted to do. I stopped her. So you know that you want to be a doctor, but you actually do not know *why* you want that career? She stared back at me. "I guess not . . . I don't know." At the end of the program Mindy decided to take a gap year and delay applying. She was prepared but not ready. She had the wisdom to recognize the difference between the two.

When I was in middle school I thought I wanted to go into medicine. I volunteered at a local hospital once a week for two years. What I discovered about myself was that I do not like sick people—at all. My ideal day at work does not include sick people or people who are in pain. As a parent and partner, I can barely deal with my loved ones who are ill. It stresses me out! Oh, and bodily fluids are a total deal breaker! Need I say more? I remember a pulmonologist and a gastroenterologist arguing once about which was more gross—sputum or stool. I had absolutely nothing to add to that conversation except that both are horrible. Had I not taken the time to explore what exactly medicine involves, hands-on, I may have fallen in love with the *idea* of medicine rather than the reality of medicine.

Your application will be stronger if you are in love with medicine in real life, not the fictitious version where everyone who needs care is beautiful and well groomed, and everyone is saved by the person in the white coat at the end of the episode. Before you invest more than eight years of your life you ought to explore your options. Doing this intentionally and with an open mind will help you identify your strengths and discern whether or not medicine is right for you. Seeking experiences that will help you explore this interest is critical. I often ask applicants to tell me something that surprised them or something that was unexpected about an experience. One student shared the following story when I asked her the question.

Shanika

I volunteered at the free clinic thinking I was helping people. I wanted to feel good at the end of the day. There were so many days I was frustrated with the system, the lack of resources, and the very limited help we were able to provide. Yes, we were providing care, but it was far from meeting the need out there. Because the clinic is so busy, patients are only allowed to pick one chief complaint during their appointment. One! Some of them have so many health issues that it's heartbreaking that we don't have more time for them. I also was surprised at how mean or angry some patients were. My bias and my ignorance to the struggles of folk who lack access to quality care caused me to expect people to be grateful and gracious all the time. We do have many patients who are this way, but we also have patients who are angry, frustrated, hurting, and marginalized. Sometimes that comes out toward us. I learned that if I am to be of service I cannot be expecting a pat on the back. I cannot be there for my own satisfaction; it's not the patient's job to be thankful or to help me be fulfilled. My job is to provide the best service and care that I can, to every patient no matter what.

Shanika was in love with medicine in real life.

Lastly, I have worked with students over the years who fell in love with the idea of themselves working in medicine and who constructed their identities around becoming a doctor. Even when receiving direct feedback and personal evidence over a long period of time that they should pursue something else they would not let go or adapt their goals.

James

I met with James, a nontraditional student in his early forties, at a premedical fair. He had been accepted to an early assurance program right out of undergrad school many years earlier. Life presented a series of challenges and he left medical school after a year. He was working in healthcare and supporting his family. He said he wanted to revisit his dream of becoming a doctor. I asked him to tell me why. He said,

I see so much disease and health ignorance in my community. I want to teach people how to take care of themselves and how to eat healthier. We need to exercise and make it central to our culture. I want to provide awareness of health issues and work to enact interventions that will improve health on a large scale. My community is suffering from poor health, and the lack of knowledge is something I am passionate about addressing.

After listening for ten minutes as he explained his purpose and goals, I pointed out that these aims were related to medicine but could be accomplished through several alternative educational and professional pathways. His goals did not require an MD degree at all, and they could be achieved more efficiently and effectively with another program. James was interested in public health, epidemiology, community activism, and nutrition. He seemed defeated when I said that doctors really don't provide health education or nutrition counseling. This is what I mean when I say he fell in love with the idea of himself working in medicine and was fixated on it. There were many viable pathways to his stated goals that were more direct, less expensive, and more closely aligned. James was locked on the idea of himself as a doctor, rather than truly exploring viable pathways for his interests, passions, and goals.

Now let me make it clear: I am not the kind of dean that discourages people. Far from it. I am a very make-it-happen-and-support-your-dreams kind of dean. If we have to make a five-year plan that's what we'll do! I once met with a student who came to me with 2.1 grade point average (GPA) and endless passion for a career in medicine. We talked truthfully about what it would take and made an extensive plan covering academic coursework, research, and engagement in healthcare. I was clear that it would take years. That student is now about to graduate from medical school having matched into a very competitive surgical sub-specialty.

Discerning Your Career Choice

There are situations where a person needs to look at all factors and seriously determine if a medical career is a good fit for their life and end goals. When I am counseling students, I ask them what elements of being a physician attract them to the profession. If they have struggled to gain admission, we then discuss what other careers have these elements that they have identified as important in their chosen line of work. Ultimately, being able to use your talents to improve the lives of others is a laudable goal. If you choose something that is not the right fit and you struggle, you will be less effective at achieving your ultimate goal, or you may not get there at all.

As you engage in preparation, pay attention to what challenges you, what excites you, and where you are successful. What feedback are you getting about your performance and preparation? Does it feel forced or natural? Is it constantly hard, or is it getting easier? It is all well and good for you to be fixated on medicine and in love with the idea that you'll be a doctor, but if you cannot find a way to make the admissions committee share that love, you won't be successful.

Medicine is a calling, not a job. It is a way of life, not a career. You will do more than earn an MD degree in medical school— you will *become* a physician. Admissions committees pay attention to motivation. If you don't really want it, medical school is the worst place to be. Allopathic medical schools in the United States have a 95 percent graduation rate, the highest graduation rate of any graduate or professional degree program out there. I must tell you, most of the time when someone doesn't finish medical school it is because of three things. In order, from the most to the least number of cases, they are 1) maturity and professionalism issues, 2) motivation issues, usually tough circumstances that produce life changes and lead to decreased motivation, and 3) academic issues. Notice that academic issues are last. We rarely dismiss people because they cannot cut it academically. Usually if they end up dismissed or voluntarily withdrawn it is initially because of maturity and motivation issues.

You must understand that if you are dismissed or withdraw from an MD program, the odds of you being able to reapply and start again later are slim to none. Very few allopathic medical schools in the United States allow applications from candidates who have previously matriculated to medical school but did not finish. You have to be ready to succeed if offered a seat.

An admissions committee does not want to give a seat to someone who may not graduate. We are sad when contemplating the tens of thousands of dollars in debt that two or three years of medical school will accrue. It breaks our hearts when someone falls short of the MD and has a tremendous loan burden that they cannot easily repay. This is why we are so careful to examine motivation and preparation on the front end.

Spend time exploring medicine in real life. Find ways to engage by volunteering, working, seeking allied health profession credentials, and/or shadowing doctors. Over the years my students have gained exposure and affirmation through medical assisting, nursing assisting, phlebotomy, patient transport, clinical research, EMT training, and dietetics. There are ways to gain proximal access to the healthcare environment so that you can confirm your motivation and expand your views of medicine. Another great way to affirm your motivation is by reading blogs, books, or scholarly articles about medicine, or listening to podcasts. Be intentional about interrogating this career choice. If you change your mind that's totally okay, and better to know sooner than later. If you affirm your decision through an active process of exploration and reflection, you will have more to write about when you apply down the road.

6

Dump the Checklist Mindset

If your prehealth adviser or premed club rep gave you a checklist, or if you found a nice "how to get into med school guide" online, now would be the time to make sure your mindset does not become focused on checking things off that list. It is important to be a well-rounded applicant and to show motivation, achievement, and exploration of medicine, but *the accumulation of experiences of a specific variety and type will not ultimately be what gets you into medical school.* The person you become as you intentionally choose experiences for your own growth and development will be the magic that sets you above the rest. You can't fake authenticity or maturity. Students often ask me, "If I have 1,000 hours of service does that look good? How many shadowing hours do I need?" The answer is not in the quantity but in the learning and development you gain. The answer is always, "It depends."

Tua

I was doing a mock interview with Tua, using his AMCAS (American Medical College Application Service) application to probe his experiences further, as many interviewers do in some way. I asked him to tell me what he learned while volunteering at a Veterans Administration (VA) nursing home for the past two years. He started to answer the question and fumbled. Then he paused our interview and said, "I actually really hated that experience. The staff were mean to me and the residents were not well cared for. I felt like they didn't want me there and I can't think of anything I want to share in an interview about it."

I paused, "Then why in the world did you volunteer there for two years?"

He replied, "Well, I needed service hours for my med school application." Yikes! Full stop. So now what? I don't recommend including anything in your application that you do not wish to openly discuss in an interview. So now this applicant was faced with a decision: risk not being able to speak openly and honestly about something he spent a lot of time doing or have a void in his application. This is why I say dump the mindset that says it is all about the checklist.

If you want to be authentic on your application, then your pursuits en route to medicine need to also be authentic. It breaks down to something my parents told me a long time ago: Do the right thing for the right reason. If your focus is on growth and development, which means making meaningful contributions in the world, you ought not to loathe the service hours you are putting in. I do not want my doctors to approach their work with obligation, regret, and a minimalist attitude. As a patient, I hope I am not merely a checklist. I would like my physicians to enjoy what they are doing, be content in their role, and be in medicine for the right reasons.

The real loss in this example is that Tua could have chosen something meaningful, personally fulfilling, and something that better used his time and gifts. He could have enjoyed connections or improved something. He missed the point. Total hours are not enough. What you took away and what you left behind are what matters. Did you take away some lessons and insights? Did you leave behind biases and self-doubt? You could volunteer at a homeless shelter for 1,000 hours, but if I ask you about that experience and you say "all homeless people are mentally ill" or "poor people just need to work hard," then it is clear that the amount of hours you performed did not yield personal learning and insight that may help you better connect with and treat patients who are experiencing homelessness. The person you become en route to my door is what matters the most.

If we shift our focus from doing the right stuff to *becoming the right person* the rules of the game change. We generate a new checklist that we make for ourselves. What kind of person do I want to be? What do I need to learn, explore, and figure out before I embark on this journey? What's my "why"? What change do I wish to see in the world and how can I become a part of that change? What are my talents and gifts? How can I apply them as I prepare myself for medicine? How do I know that this career direction is right for me?

Application Inflation

Another symptom of the checklist mentality is that it causes people to inflate their experiences and embellish their hours. Applicants are tempted to present their experiences in a way that makes what they did count for the checklist. There are only twenty-four hours in a day, so please, for the love of logic, do not list experiences with hours that exceed this maximum. If you say you did something for twelve months, you cannot list 6,570 hours. That would mean you only slept six hours a night for an entire year and every other waking minute you were working. You never showered, ate, shopped for food, or traveled to and from your job? We can add and multiply, so don't exaggerate. Quality over quantity, my friends.

I once had an applicant indicate on his application that he had won an Oscar. Wow, impressive! I looked up the film and did not find his name anywhere in the credits. This applicant was in our summer program, so I asked him about the experience. "Can I see your Oscar statue?" I asked. He was a little embarrassed to admit he did not have one. He said he had volunteered for two weeks as an interpreter to travel with the film crew for a few of the interviews that had taken place outside the United States. He had a friend who was connected to the film crew, so the applicant was fortunate to have the opportunity to participate in a documentary about human rights.

I helped the applicant rewrite an accurate description of the experience and his involvement with the project, including that the film went on to win an Oscar. If he had submitted the embellished version it may have actually taken away from the experience and interviewers may have been disappointed to hear that he didn't actually have an Oscar from the Academy of Motion Picture Arts and Sciences. An accurate description explained his involvement in an experience that was something genuinely impressive.

When you agree to the terms and submit your application, you are attesting to the truthfulness of everything in it. Your integrity as a future professional matters right now. While applicants may think they will be more competitive putting more hours down or claiming something was service when it was not, these inaccuracies typically bleed through. It is the meaning-making and the personal gains from your experiences that truly create value, not the hours. The hours you cataloged likely will not compensate for gaps in reflection and depth in both initial and subsequent phases of the admissions process.

Copycat Syndrome

I often see applications from students from the same undergraduate institution that seem to follow a template. Students have largely participated in the same extracurricular and enrichment activities. They chose the same clubs and service endeavors, locally and globally. Their letters of recommendation are from the same professors. The application writing is safe and sterile, usually summarizing the experiences all over again. These applicants come from well-structured schools with good premed resources and connections.

While there is nothing wrong with using the resources of your premed advising office, you should recognize that following a prescribed path is not likely to yield experiences (or an application) that will help you stand out to admissions committees.

Begin with Passion

Standing out as a unique and well-rounded applicant begins with passion. Do what you love; love what you do. It really is that simple. If you are exploring your career and seeking experiences that will help you discern medicine, you will cover the needed bases to find your why. If you let your passion and interests guide your pursuits, you will have a much higher likelihood of being successful. And as a bonus, you will enjoy the journey much more as well.

Cassie

Cassie wanted to stretch herself by doing research and was struggling to find something for a summer semester. She had a small grant for a research program and could work with any faculty member that would take her on as a mentee. She had a few meetings with cancer biologists, clinical researchers, and an endocrinologist, but none of the projects really spoke to her. She didn't want to be in a lab all day.

In her spare time Cassie loved to skateboard. She rode her board around campus and frequently went to skate parks. I mentioned that there was an exercise and sports science department on campus and she should ask around there if they were undertaking any research related to sports. Eventually Cassie found a faculty member who studied sports injuries and proposed a project examining different types of helmets and the levels of protection they provided to skateboarders. She spent time sending dummy models through the halfpipe at the local skate park to mimic certain types of falls and measured the energy transfer of the falls through sensors in the helmets. Ultimately, she enjoyed her summer, she accomplished her goal of doing research, and she learned more than she expected about equation modeling, where knowledge comes from, and field research. If you ask her about her project she will still talk about it with enthusiasm. She was able to get a strong letter of recommendation from the faculty member with whom she worked because her performance was excellent for the project. Her passion led the way for success. Had she chosen something about which she was not passionate, she may not have been able to get a strong letter of recommendation. (And she certainly would have had considerably less fun that summer.)

If your application could be quantified into buckets of how you spent your time during your premed years, what categories would that time fall under? Do the categories and quantities reflect your values? Do they reflect your ultimate goals in medicine? The best way to tell a committee who you are is to show them. What you claim has to be backed up with action in your application and reflection in your interview. Begin with passion and your identity will come through authentically. Don't be boxed in by convention or what you think is the mold. The experience does not matter more than the takeaway does.

Mikayla

Another of my student interviews was Mikayla. Her family owned a small diner and she had worked there her entire life and throughout college, first washing dishes on a milk crate in the back kitchen, then becoming a server and eventually assistant manager. I asked her what the restaurant industry taught her. She blew me away with her insights about her experience.

It takes a ton of intelligence and savvy to run a restaurant. The timing, teamwork, and coordination make all the difference in success or failure. The cooks have to work well with the servers, and the bussers have to get along with everyone, too. Management has to value every person equally. It is not enough for each person to understand their role; they must also understand how their role affects the roles of others on the team. The best team members not only do their job but allow others to do their jobs well also.

According to Mikayla,

The most salient thing I learned is that often the most important piece of information you need to help someone effectively they usually will not tell you directly. Customers will often not tell you what you need to do to meet their expectations. You have to observe their behavior and figure it out. You have to give them permission to share by how you ask. If I have a customer order scrambled eggs with cheese and I notice that they took one bite and did not eat them, I have all the information I need to provide better service. They ordered [scrambled eggs] specifically . . . , they planned to eat them, and something went wrong. I do not casually ask, "How is everything?" as I brisk by, or "Are the eggs OK?" while I pour coffee. I pause and make direct eye contact and I say, "It looks like our eggs didn't meet your expectations. What can I get you instead? When I bring you new ones, what should we do differently?" Customers will take me up on this offer every time. I give them permission to let me help them without being afraid that I'm mad or someone will think they are a pain.

I have noticed this as a teaching assistant at school, too. My students often don't say what it is that they need the most, but I can anticipate that need and approach them in a way that provides an open door for them to get what they need. I know some students need additional help, so I say, "What day and time works for supplemental instruction this week?" not "Do you need supplemental instruction this week?" Usually the ones who need help suggest the times and get what they need. I've learned that this makes a huge difference in being able to help effectively.

Clearly, Mikayla is a student who is paying attention and who has grown from her experiences. She learned more about effective interaction with her future patients by working in a diner than some others do working in a clinic. When Mikayla and I met, she was initially worried that the time she spent working would take away from her candidacy because the work wasn't medically related. Far from it. She had gained so much by meaningfully contributing to her family's business and supporting herself through school. She could talk about teamwork, commitment, taking responsibility, accountability, conflict resolution, and people skills with ease. She readily shared her life experiences and her character absolutely shined through. She is the kind of person I would want for my future doctor.

7

The Secret to a Competitive Edge

Students often ask me what my school is looking for, how to stand out, and how to be competitive in the process. They are seeking something that can give them a competitive edge. What is the special ingredient that will help you be competitive? Well, first it is recognizing that you are a human being, not a human doing. What you *do* is only relevant if it is genuinely connected to who you *are*. Your pursuits should be anchored to your authentic self, otherwise you are floating about on the ocean with no real direction. If we cannot tell where you are going, it's hard for us to tell if you will be a good fit for our institution. *The secret to a competitive edge is growth.* You should take time to reflect on your personal growth: independence, resilience, determination, and challenges that have tested you.

So how do we grow? It's an odd question, but I am being serious. What do we do if we realize that we need to grow more before applying to medical school? The growth zone exists where you are uncomfortable or vulnerable, working hard, and paying attention. The possibility of failure is real in the growth zone. To grow a muscle you have to stretch it and actually break it down a little. Such is true with our characters and true selves.

Dana

Dana grew up in a rural town in Idaho. She attended a state school and stayed close to family. She decided to apply for AmeriCorps in order to experience a different life setting and a different population.

As a volunteer she lived and worked in an urban setting in the Midwest. She tutored youth at a school that was predominantly Latino and where the graduation rate was below 40 percent. She developed relationships with her fellow corps members who were very different from her. Although it was not easy, Dana loved what she was doing. She spent an additional year as a senior corps member because she enjoyed it so much. During her time she kept a journal where she reflected on her biases weekly and wrote down experiences that were meaningful or challenging to her. She actively questioned her thinking and assumptions many times. She gained new perspectives about her upbringing and her identity. Not only did her time volunteering help her grow, it also strengthened her personally in confidence, interpersonal skills, independence, resilience—all these areas improved because she chose to do something that challenged her while also giving back.

Connect across Difference

Another secret to having a competitive edge is the ability to connect across differences. We tend to be very invested in our comfort zones—that is, we choose to surround ourselves by like-minded people. I often see applications that indicate the candidates have a lot of engagement with many facets of one organization or community. This is wonderful, but when all the experiences are insular to the same environment, committee members are left wondering about adaptability, resilience, and relationship skills. It is easy to get along with like-minded people with whom you are comfortable. Reaching across differences builds empathy and maturity. Encountering people and situations that are different may produce discomfort and an element of failure, but it is a strong indicator of growth.

Becca

Becca was a runner. She loved to run and did so daily. She saw a flyer advertising for volunteer runner guides for runners with low vision. It piqued her curiosity, so she signed up. She learned how to describe the terrain and to time her descriptions appropriately for various paces. She gained real insight into how visually impaired individuals navigate the world that she could not have understood without firsthand experience. The biggest thing she told me that she learned was that people are very proud of their communities, and they do not live their lives thinking they have a deficit. She realized that she previously had a bias about individuals with disabilities, that she felt sorry for them. Those feelings, she later came to understand, were more about her own discomfort than anything else. I asked Becca if anyone ever fell when she was guiding them.

Yes. And the first time it happened I felt really awful. My companion runner, Toby, was a great sport about the whole thing. As we started running again he showed me great kindness as he could tell I was very hesitant and afraid. He said, "We can't run together if you're afraid. You're the one who can see. We both have to rely on you." Toby taught me that he defines being disabled as allowing something to limit you or hold you back. In many areas in life he isn't "disabled" at all. That day I almost allowed my fear to hold us back, so it turned out that I was the one who was really "disabled" that day.

So there you have it. That's the sweet spot—find something you love and figure out how to make someone's life better doing it. Get outside yourself and see what you find. You should hopefully take insights with you and leave behind biases, fears, and insecurity.

Systems-Based Thinking

Another ingredient in the competitive edge is understanding structures and systems. Learning to think beyond your current circumstance and to see situations from another perspective is a critical skill in medicine. As you approach your experiences, use a systems-based lens to drive your learning and reflection. We want to see your critical-thinking skills. We need to know that you can reflect more deeply than "helping people feels good" or "science is exciting." When you understand the interaction of people and systems, you become an applicant that stands out.

Take time to create a systems web of your experiences. This means identifying all the related systems and issues and seeking greater understanding. This is one of the best ways to prepare for an interview because through your learning you will strengthen and deepen your reflection and understanding of the context of your experiences. Your conversations then take on more meaning and relevance. Consider Tua's example of volunteering at a nursing home run by the VA (see chapter 6). What does the systems web look like? There are countless ways to explore these complex interconnected issues and systems. Begin with brainstorming the areas that you have observed in both people and systems interactions and build from there. How does it function? What are its strengths and weaknesses? What news stories are there about the system or its people? What do the people working in the system think of it? Curiosity is a critical tool in growth and reflection—it means you are paying attention. How do systems interact with each other? What are the results of these intersections? Consider interactions at the personal, familial, community, local, and global levels. Examine government/policy, health outcomes, health disparities, healthcare access, and cultural impacts. If you observe differences, explore them to understand them. Figure 7.1 is an example of how we might sketch out a simple systems web to channel curiosity and promote learning (see following). The related areas in this example are aging issues, grief and loss, staff challenges, policies, VA healthcare, veteran health, and caregivers.

Next, expand your systems web by brainstorming related areas of the experience or issues on each node. Figure 7.2 is an example of an expanded systems web with related topics and ideas on each node (see following).

For the aging issues node we might expand that with more specific subtopics to explore ethics and shared decision making, end

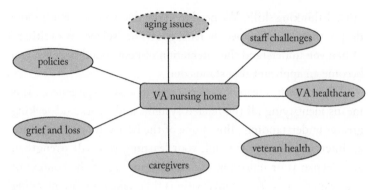

FIG. 7.1 Basic Systems Web

of life care, independence and autonomy, income changes and retirement, and cultural issues (see figure 7.3). The veteran health node (not shown) could be populated with subtopics such as mental health, physical health, rehabilitation and disabilities, professional occupations and employment programs, effects of trauma, and disparities. Move through each node identifying subtopics, expanding as many times as needed to accommodate relationships and ideas. Once you have completed topics for each stem, you will have a guide for independent learning and inquiry that also helps conceptualize how the ideas are related. Begin learning more by seeking articles, podcasts, organizations, and other resources to expand your knowledge and understanding.

Here is another example of how we can think about systems. When I was in graduate school I had a friend in my classes who had been through hard times. Julie often shared her struggles with past addiction, homelessness, and trauma. She gave us all the gift of candor and vulnerability in the classroom. Julie heard me talking one day about my medical students planning a health fair. She entered the conversation by saying, "So what, exactly, is accomplished by this so-called health fair?" She had a high degree of sarcasm in her tone.

I said, "Well, the students will do blood pressure and glucose screenings. They plan to have some information about nutrition with free samples and grocery coupons. A few of them are yoga

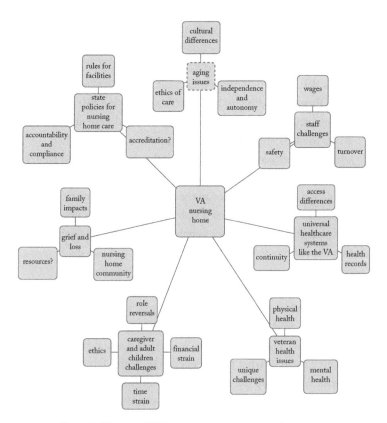

FIG. 7.2 Expanded Systems Web

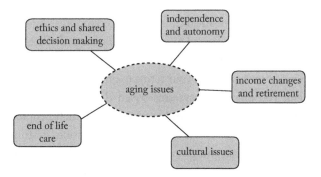

FIG. 7.3 Systems Web Subtopics

teachers and want to do free yoga as part of the fair." Julie recoiled and said,

> That's BS. I've been to those events before. I didn't have health-care. They did nothing to help me. So when I find that my blood pressure and blood sugar are high, then what? I have no doctor or access to medication. When I learn how to eat healthy, then what? I eat whatever they hand out at the shelter, the food pantry, or the dollar menu if I have a dollar. Discount coupons are useless if you don't have any money in the first place. Do you actually think education helps when people are starving? And yoga! Do you actually think that poor people are interested in yoga? We don't have time, space, or money for uppity stuff like that!

Julie was right to criticize our efforts. My students and I had not really engaged in systems-based thinking to examine why the people we claimed we were trying to help were situated on the margins in the first place. In fact, we hadn't even asked them how we could serve them or what they needed. The health fair was our idea, not theirs. Why were they poor? What did they need? If we truly wanted to help, what should we do? I am surprised how infrequently those that are comfortably seated on the benches fail to ask the folk in the trenches about their perspectives. If you want to get outside your comfort zone, you have to get off the bench, get a new view, aim to critically think about your beliefs, why you have them, and ultimately confront some biases and blind spots. The students' ideas about health were not invalid, but they were poorly aligned with what the people they desired to serve actually needed. Therefore the service was more about the students than the people they wanted to help. Service exclusively on your terms mainly serves you.

When you engage in systems-based thinking you step back and examine the structures and systems with which people interact to determine larger issues that result in oppression, dysfunction, disenfranchisement, and poor outcomes. Even the interventions and proposed solutions should be part of this analysis. Do they work? How do they work? Who designed them? If they work well, why? If they do not work well, why not? If you want to be a next-level applicant, you absolutely must do this kind of analysis. For each experience that you have, do a systems-level analysis and work to understand the interrelationships of the issues. The more you learn about these areas, the better prepared you will be to engage in meaningful discussions about your experience. Systems-based thinking coupled with personal reflection on meaning is the best interview preparation.

Jared

Jared taught self-defense classes at the YWCA. He volunteered regularly and enjoyed sharing his skills (he was a black belt in taekwondo) with members of the community. The first few months after he started teaching, I asked him how it was going. He said, "I'm having a lot of fun. I really like empowering women and giving them tools to stay safe." I challenged him a little.

"For the next few months I would like for you to begin your class by asking your participants why they are taking your class and what they hope to gain." He agreed. Two months later Jared checked in with me about his time at the YWCA. He said,

> I cannot believe how unsafe the world is for women compared to men. I have heard so many stories of fear and even assault. I always sort of knew this happened, but I never thought about it *personally*. Women feel unsafe in various situations every single day. I totally take for granted that as a man I almost never feel unsafe. We don't market self-defense classes to men. Then I started to realize that most assaults are perpetrated by men and I'm thinking, "What can I do to make the world safer for women so they don't have to take a self-defense class in the first place? How come we don't ask men to take classes where they learn to look out for and defend women, or to not assault women in the first place?"
>
> Then I realized that there are tons of ways I experience the world that I take for granted based on things I don't control, like my skin color, my social class, my education. And now I'm

overwhelmed thinking "What do I do now?" There's so much that needs to change.

I had a wonderful discussion with Jared about using his privilege to be an ally, and we had a long conversation about the personal commitments he was willing to make. When he began at the YWCA he showed up and he was committed. He was sharing his talents and giving his time. That was great. But it was only when he started listening and paying attention that he was really able to see the systems in play that influenced the world around him. He was then able to see how these systems influenced the women he was serving. The insight he gained from the experience is more powerful and demonstrative of his strengths than simply volunteering. Becoming a leader, change agent, and ally are wonderful aspects of preparation in medicine. I'd like my doctor to be all three.

Learning to Lead

A fourth ingredient in the competitive edge is learning to lead. Physicians are the leaders of the healthcare team. They must learn to be leaders and good team members. What does it mean to lead? How do you develop leadership skills? We are looking for you to be in charge of more than just yourself. We like to see evidence of your ability to collaborate and work well with others. Learning to lead means building skills, not collecting titles. Leadership comes in many forms. It isn't always being the president of something; it's also a process. As you challenge yourself and learn to lead, pay attention. Again, I encourage you to choose things that you are passionate about and pursue areas where you would like to create impact and change.

Ezra

Ezra was a second year undergraduate. He had played football throughout high school and stayed connected with his high school team. He was volunteering in his spare time to help coach practices for the ninth-grade team twice a week. I asked him what he had learned as a coach. I loved his insights about leadership.

When I first started running practices, it was sort of a disaster. The guys didn't respect me and they wouldn't really listen or work hard for me. There was a lot of goofing around and talking over my instructions. I was frustrated and went to my former coach, the varsity coach, for advice. He asked to review my practice plans. I didn't have any. He asked to review my individual skill reports on my players. I didn't have any. He asked what team goals we had set for the season. I didn't have an answer for that, either.

My coach helped me see that I wasn't taking practice very seriously and the guys could see that. If I wanted their respect, I'd have to earn it by investing in them and showing them I was also working hard. As I began planning, working with players individually and setting team goals, everything changed. We eventually established team values that we went over at every team meeting. I learned so much during my time coaching. All my life I have taken good leadership for granted. Now I really see that effective leaders work harder than their followers. They take greater responsibility for outcomes than everyone else. They understand that respect is earned. When things aren't going well, effective leaders rely on values to inform their behavior.

Ezra did not have a glamorous title as president, founder, or CEO. He was a volunteer ninth-grade football coach, but the insights he gained about leadership demonstrated his preparation in that area. Talking to Ezra you would get the idea that he understands the qualities of a leader and how to be effective. He is also someone I would want on my team.

Let's review the components of the competitive edge:

1. Growth. Get outside the comfort zone and challenge yourself. Reflect on your experiences and what they mean.
2. Connect across difference. Challenge your biases. Get uncomfortable.

3. Engage in systems-based thinking. Apply a critical lens and curiosity to your experiences and deepen your understanding.
4. Learn to lead. Recognize that there are many opportunities for leadership development if we view leadership as a process rather than a position.

Now that we are done talking about preparation for the premed journey, let's talk about making the application.

PART III

Advice for Application Season

8

The Inside Scoop on Strategy and Maximizing Mission Fit

Every year there is at least one person who applies to every single school through the American Medical College Application Service (AMCAS). I do not recommend this. How do you figure out where to apply? How do you know if a school is a good fit for you? You absolutely need an application strategy, and it begins with knowing yourself. Assess your strengths and limitations as an applicant. Determine your goals in medicine and the qualities and characteristics you wish to gain through your medical education. Do your homework and research schools. Go online and learn all you can about prospective schools and their missions. Do not apply to schools about which you know nothing. Spend time researching the process at the schools you are interested in and pay special attention to their missions.

Here's an important fact: You can't be all things to all schools. If you try to squeeze into every school's mold, you are going to lose all the flair that makes you who you are. You will come across as a generic applicant that is trying to fit a mold. Remember, the best applicants are authentic and self-aware. You will need to determine which schools are a good fit for your strengths and which ones have missions that you feel align with your own. Present yourself confidently and authentically to maximize your odds.

The application window spans several months, but the consideration applicants receive is greatest at the beginning of the cycle. You want to be in early! Most schools employ a rolling admissions process. What does that mean? It means that when the season opens they begin reviewing files and moving them along to the next phase. Interview seats begin to fill and acceptances are issued beginning October 15. This is the earliest date for offers that is agreed on by all AMCAS participating schools (except those with early admission programs). If you are submitting your application in October, the likelihood that a school has an opportunity to give it the same consideration as the application submitted in July or August is slim. Every season there are applicants who are not considered because time runs out. Schools always try to do their best to read as many files as possible. One of my schools, for example, conducted more than 10,000 reviews during the 2017–2018 cycle and there were still some files we were unable to thoroughly screen.

The "apply early" advice comes with a caveat. An early application of poor quality will not benefit you. If you are not ready or your application is sloppy, being early will not make up the difference. Therefore I am advising you to manage the timing of your application well so that you can plan to apply in the beginning months of the cycle to maximize your chances. You need to be flexible and you need to plan ahead. The AMCAS application usually opens May 1, and the cycle opens June 1, which is the earliest date applications can be submitted. Schools typically do not begin downloading files until around July 1. There is a lag because we are still finalizing our classes from the cycle before, which doesn't end until the first day of school for the new class. Although start dates vary, they are mainly late July and early August for most schools.

Pro Tip: You can find the orientation and start dates for all schools in the Medical School Admission Requirements (MSAR) Online.[1] If you are obsessing about applying exactly on June 1, you can relax a little. If you apply June 10, my school will likely get your application at the same time as if you applied June 1. The AMCAS verification team is efficient, and although the time allotted for verification is weeks, it can happen in a few days.

The Cost of Applying

Applying is expensive. The average applicant will spend $3,500 to apply through AMCAS and complete supplemental applications to twenty schools. This total does not include the costs of traveling to interviews. You absolutely need to plan ahead so that finances will not limit how you engage the process as an applicant. The Association of American Medical Colleges (AAMC) has a Fee Assistance Program (FAP)[2] for applicants who qualify. You can go to the website and use a preliminary calculator that will tell you if you meet the guidelines. The FAP waiver is good for eighteen months, and it is not retroactive. You must obtain the FAP waiver before you register and pay for any services. In addition to waiving the cost of applying to up to twenty schools, the FAP provides a reduced Medical College Admission Test (MCAT) fee, MSAR Online access for free, and some discounted or free MCAT preparation materials as well.

Most schools will honor the FAP waiver for supplemental applications either automatically or by request, so obtaining the waiver can greatly reduce your total cost. If you were not able to obtain the FAP waiver you can still be proactive and request a supplemental waiver from schools by reaching out via email and providing an explanation and documentation. Most admissions deans do not want circumstances or financial barriers to limit applicants, and you should look into the policies for supplemental waivers at each school. If it will stretch your dollar, it's worth asking. Also note that processing supplemental fee waivers may delay your application slightly, so ask up front.

If you have a limited budget, make sure you consider the cost at each phase. It is not efficient to apply to twenty schools through AMCAS if you cannot afford to complete the supplemental applications. Only complete applications can be considered for admission. If you do not plan to complete an application at a school, it is a waste of money to apply there. Examine your budget and develop a strategy that is within those constraints. If you feel your budget does not allow you to apply to enough schools, address that issue before you apply. If relatives and friends ask what you would like for your birthday or a holiday, ask them to contribute to your medical school application fund. Begin financially planning for the application process so that you are able to maximize the opportunity for consideration.

Every Process Is Different

Each time I speak with an admissions colleague I am amazed at the variety of admissions processes out there. No two are alike, quite literally. There are different structures and decision-making strategies at each school. All of them include faculty. All of them include a concrete set of guidelines that a school aims to efficiently, fairly, and universally apply. There are some basic elements you can deduce from the MSAR data from the AAMC. One important element is whether the school is public or private. Public schools are more likely to have a preference for state residents, which can impact the admissions process. Another is whether files are screened prior to supplemental invitations being extended. Many schools send supplemental invitations to everyone and thus do not screen until files are complete. There are some schools that only invite a select group to complete a supplemental. At these schools receiving an invitation for a supplemental means you have cleared review already, at least preliminarily.

Supplemental fees and deadlines also vary by institution. Some schools give you a deadline specific to your invitation—say, forty-five days. Some schools have a universal deadline that all applicants must meet regardless of when they were invited to complete an application. If a school specifies a deadline, it is critical to meet that deadline or you risk discontinuing your candidacy. Admissions at most schools are rolling, so no matter the supplemental deadline you should complete your application as soon as possible. Fees may also vary by school. Some schools allow you to view and work on the application and ask for the fee upon submission. Other schools require you pay a fee up front in order to obtain access to the supplemental. In these instances you pay the fee regardless of whether you complete the application. Fees range, with the average being about $100 per school.

MCAT Tips

There are a few things about the MCAT that you need to know in advance. 1) Scores are forever, 2) timing matters, and 3) don't miss the head fake.

SCORES ARE FOREVER

Every time you take the MCAT and confirm that you would like it to be scored, the scores are recorded under your AAMC ID number. This number is the same number you will use when you apply for medical school through AMCAS. The scores will automatically be visible on your AMCAS application and you cannot withhold or hide scores to schools. We see all your scored attempts along with the dates you took the exams. We may even see scores that are no longer within the date range for eligible scores.

Here's an important tip that I wish more applicants knew about: When you sit for the MCAT, the test gives you an option to void your test at the end. This means that your test will not be scored and there will be no record that you attempted it. You will never know the score and neither will we. I do not recommend using this option liberally, but if you know you had a bad test day you should consider it. What is a bad test day? Obviously it's subjective, but a few examples might be not finishing the sections, guessing on an inordinate number of questions, being distracted by illness or another condition, having an extremely high level of anxiety, or dealing with a testing center issue (e.g., a power outage, fire alarm). If you choose to void your test you will not receive a refund. Nonetheless, I think it is important to share this tip because many students do not pay attention to this option at the end and tell me that they knew they did poorly but opted to have the exam scored anyway.

TIMING MATTERS

You will want to make sure that you schedule your exam in advance so that you can get the date range you planned. Seats usually fill quickly at the testing centers around the country. Also, be aware that you cannot be scheduled for more than one exam at a time, so you must wait until your test date in order to schedule another attempt. This means that if your time line includes a July test date, you will not receive your scores until August. If you are unhappy with your scores and wish to sit again, testing dates for the season may be full or may be too far into the fall to have a timely application.

The AMCAS application reports whether you have a pending MCAT score. At most schools if you indicate a pending score, your application is held until that score is released. Some schools have minimum cutoffs and will forward your file with a pending score if your current application meets that minimum, but that's rare. So understand that even if you applied early, if you choose to retake the MCAT during the cycle you are delaying your file and may be negating an early submission date. If you think you may need more than one attempt at the MCAT, plan for that. Better to anticipate and plan for that scenario than find yourself rushing to retake it during the cycle and incurring delay. Do not let timing be an X factor that you don't anticipate. If you end up reapplying, it will be hard to deduce how much of the outcome was related to timing and how much was your application itself.

DON'T MISS THE HEAD FAKE

The MCAT can be a significant barrier for many applicants. Depending on your previous relationship with standardized exams, you may anticipate the test with confidence or a high degree of anxiety. Take the time to address your test-taking skills and strategies during your preparation. Many applicants mistakenly think that if they could only get a decent enough MCAT, they will get into medical school and live happily ever after. Nope. The head fake is this: If you desire to be a practicing physician you are signing up for a lifetime of standardized exams. The MCAT is the *first* hurdle, and certainly not the last. The more you prepare and build a strong skill set for succeeding on exams, the better off you will be in medical school and beyond. During all your years of medical school you will take tests. There will be exams on basic science material as well as clinical knowledge exams related to different medical specialties. You will also need to complete the United States Medical Licensing Examination (USMLE)[3] to become a licensed physician in the United States. USMLE has multiple steps: Step 1, Step 2 Clinical Skills, Step 2 Clinical Knowledge, and Step 3. Steps 1 and 2 are taken during medical school and are required to graduate. Step 3 is usually taken following the first year of residency. Many residency programs have exams at various training checkpoints to benchmark milestones and learning objectives; these are called *in-training exams*. If you wish to become board certified in your specialty, you will need to complete a board exam at the end of residency. You will also have to recertify every seven to ten years depending on your specialty.

While the MCAT has varying degrees of influence on admissions across schools, it remains important because it does help committees understand your preparedness for standardized tests. While you are preparing for the MCAT, pay attention to your study skills and methods. If you take an MCAT prep course, focus on the skills as well as the content. It is not just the material you need to master, it is the entire process of learning, comprehending, and showing what you know in the format of a standardized test. Learn how you learn best so you can apply those same strategies to your future exam endeavors. Do not make the mistake of viewing the MCAT as a one-time hurdle. All your investment in test-taking skills will pay dividends in medical school and beyond.

Be Organized

You know by now that to succeed in school you need the skill sets to efficiently execute tasks and keep track of details. You need these executive-function skills more than ever in order to be a strong applicant. I have seen some impressive organizational tools used by applicants over the years: spreadsheets, online documents, expandable files, binders, color codes, etc. Whatever your method, be intentional about keeping everything straight, meeting deadlines, and maintaining solid records/logs of your progress at each school. Each school will likely have an online interface requiring a user name and password. Know what you have submitted and when. Save screenshots or your own copies of your supplemental materials. Each school will have different deadlines and requirements that you need to meet. Keep track of these as well.

Remember that the burden of proof is always on the applicant. We receive a high volume of phone calls weekly and are managing thousands of applications. You only have to manage yours. If you want to advocate for yourself, you will need to have detailed notes with dates, times, names, and so on. Keep your emails organized, too. It is always up to the applicant to ensure their file is complete and that they can meet all requirements for the school. If you are missing a letter of recommendation and that is the only outstanding element needed to complete your file, we are not going to call you to remind you. Schools do not have the capacity to keep track of student applications on a micro level. Again, we receive thousands of complete files annually. How well candidates demonstrate the ability to keep on top of their own application is also part of our screening criteria. If you cannot manage your own process of applying to medical school, we feel that you are not ready to manage the care of patients in a few short years.

Rock That Personal Statement

As I said in the preface, the idea for this book came on the heels of a piece I wrote for my department's medical education blog,

ReflectiveMedEd.org.[4] The piece is entitled *Tough Love for Your Personal Statement: Advice from a Medical School Admissions Dean.* My perspective on application writing comes from decades of reading phenomenal and impactful personal statements as well as boring and disturbing ones.

When I work with applicants I encourage them to focus on answering the "How" and "Why" questions to show the committee the depth of their experiences. Applicants frequently fall into the trap of making a lot of declarative sentences. "I know I want to work with underserved communities." How? "I am well prepared to take on the challenges of medicine." How do you know that? "I believe that healthcare is a human right." Why? Carefully review your statement and look for the declarations you have made. In every case, did you explain how and why?

Here are some questions that can get you going if you are stuck. I encourage you to write and prepare answers to any of these questions that appeal to you. Start by broadly reflecting and then try to narrow in on something that conveys your passion for medicine in a powerful way.

1. Who are the influential people in my life?
2. What are the influential elements of my life?
3. Where are my "forks" in the road?
4. How do I describe myself?
5. How do others describe me?
6. What are my hopes and dreams?
7. Why do I want to be a doctor?
8. What do I hope to accomplish in medicine? Why can't that be accomplished in another field?
9. Who are my role models?
10. What are the most important things in my life?
11. What makes me unique?
12. What gives me confidence?
13. What brings me joy?
14. What keeps me up at night?
15. What has surprised me lately?

16. What are my hobbies? Why do I like them?
17. What are the lessons I have learned in life and where did I learn them?
18. What makes me sad? Happy?
19. What does my ideal world look like?
20. How have my loved ones influenced my journey?
21. If I could change one thing about my life, what would it be? Why?
22. If I could change one thing about medicine, what would it be? Why?
23. What do I bring to medicine that others might not?
24. What assumptions do people make about me?
25. What is something about me that people could never guess?
26. What are my strengths? What are my limitations?
27. What have I learned preparing for medical school?
28. What is the greatest hardship I've faced in life?
29. What have I learned from adversity?
30. How do I respond to challenges?
31. What part of my life is unrelated to medicine?
32. What are my aspirations if I don't get into medical school? What other career would come close to offering what medicine does?
33. What is my preferred way to communicate? Why?
34. What are the elements of my culture that are most important to me? How has my culture influenced my life?
35. What about my background is visible or invisible to medicine?
36. What groups do I belong to and how have they influenced me?
37. What identities do I carry and how do those identities influence my worldview and my passion for medicine?
38. What are the pros and cons of a career in medicine?

If you engage in the process of preparing a strong personal statement, you will ultimately be able to better explain your reasons for wanting to work in medicine. You will be better prepared to confidently explain yourself and your passion to others. You should dedicate a few solid months to constructing, evaluating, and perfecting your personal statement. It is a process, not an event.

How personal is too personal? That is up to you. If you are authentic and sincere, that should come through in your message regardless of topic or focus. If you are considering sharing something in your application that you feel is controversial, ask yourself, "Is this detail critical to my motivation for medicine?" If yes, and you simply cannot discuss your journey without it, then you should work to find a way to convey that information. If not, consider choosing something unique but with less potential liabilities. Remember, we do not yet know you, so your essay gives us a window into your personhood. I have read powerful essays about abuse, neglect, and trauma. I have read essays about mental illness, infectious disease, and other maladies. I cannot generalize as to whether they are always effective or always too risky. What I can tell you is that the good ones were not asking to be admitted *because* they had suffered, they were describing their formation of motivation and compassion with a story of personal suffering as the backdrop. There is a big difference in the tone and overall feel. You must conclude and arrive at a destination by the end that leaves the reader inspired and confident about you as a person. You should also not leave the reader wondering about your health or mental state if you choose to write about something that is deeply personal.

Please note that your personal statement need not contain grand, flashy experiences or personal trauma. Do not compare yourself to others who have different motivations and experiences. You need to be authentic and explain your why. I have read amazing personal statements about seemingly mundane things, like growing up while working in a family business, learning to ski, and taking morning walks. It is the reflection of your personal growth and unique, authentic perspective that matters.

Have your friends read your personal statement. Have people that you don't know read it. Gather feedback by asking specific questions of your readers. Does this essay make you want to meet me in person? Is this essay interesting? Did this essay keep your attention throughout? Was anything distracting or concerning? What are your impressions of me after reading this statement? Do not just ask people if your essay is good. That is far too generic a question to elicit constructive feedback. Because I love you and I really want you to have a phenomenal personal statement, I am sharing with you a simple tool you can use. I call it my feedback rubric (see table 8.1). Please feel free to use it to evaluate your own work, or give it to someone from whom you are seeking feedback during your writing process.

My last tip for personal statements: Use the line test to ensure your statement is engaging. Instruct your readers that if at any point they are bored or do not wish to read further, they should draw a line across the page at that point in the essay and hand it back to you. If the essay does not engage the reader, it will not be effective in helping you get an interview. *The goal of your entire application is to compel the reviewers and decision makers to want to meet you in person.* You can only get a seat if you are first chosen for an interview.

Supplemental Writing Tips

I often get asked how important the essays or personal statements are for the admissions process. These questions are sometimes asked by applicants who are skeptical as to whether these elements of their application are ever actually read. My answer is this: If they were not important we would not ask for them. Do not ask me for permission to do the minimum or gloss over elements of the application that schools require. One of the best ways to stand out to committees is to spend the time customizing your application for their school. We ask questions in our supplemental because we

TABLE 8.1. Dean Nakae's Personal Statement Feedback Rubric

Writer's Name:_____ Reviewer's Name:_____

Date:_____

I would use the following adjectives to describe how this statement made me feel:

After reading this statement, I learned the following about the writer:

Sense of writer's passion/motivation for medicine

Generic claims about motivation. Few personal details given. No concrete, clear motivation expressed.	Some idea of motivation, but not expressed in a powerful or personal way.	Strong expression of motivation, but some clarification and fine-tuning is needed.	Strong, clear expression of motivation and passion for medicine that is deeply personal. Leaves the reader with a memorable takeaway.

Sense of writer's identity

No clear idea of who the writer is and/or where they are coming from.	Some idea of writer's identity, but ideas are sparse and/or not well developed.	Solid expression of writer's identity and background.	Solid expression of writer's identity and background *and* how it relates to their motivation/passion for medicine.

Sense of writer's self-awareness and/or self-appraisal

Writer's tone is overly confident or oblivious to self-appraisal. Unaware of self in relation to others and/or the world.	Writer's tone is distant from the subject, with little intersection of self-awareness or place in the world.	Writer's tone is self-aware and interconnected with essay content appropriately.	Writer's tone is humble, offering realistic self-appraisal and solid evidence of understanding of self in relation to others.

Point of view/empathy/perspective-taking

No evidence that the writer can engage in perspective-taking or consider alternative points of view.	Some evidence that writer can consider alternative points of view, but seems dismissive of them or self-righteous/critical of others.	Solid evidence of perspective-taking and empathy. Writer demonstrates ability and openness to engage outside of self and take on new perspectives.

Continued on page 88

TABLE 8.1. (continued)

How did the writer engage the reader?

Essay is not engaging. Reader is compelled to start skimming immediately or stop reading before reaching the end.	Essay is engaging at first but doesn't hold my attention. Scattered or too varied in topic area.	Essay is engaging and holds attention throughout.	Essay is gripping and really makes the reader want to meet the writer.

Distractions/red flags

Essay contains many distractions of superfluous details, shocking elements, or boundary concerns.	Essay has some areas that are distracting and need to be revisited or refined in the next draft.	Essay has no distractions or red flags that are disruptive to the reader.	

Grammar, sentence structure, word choice

Grammar, sentence structure, and/or word choice need considerable work.	Grammar, sentence structure, and/or word choice need some work.	Grammar, sentence structure, and/or word choice are solid—minor edits needed.	Grammar, sentence structure, and/or word choice are stellar—perfect or near perfect.

Organization/flow/transitions

Ideas did not flow logically. Ideas were difficult to follow. The essay's organization needs considerable work.	Some areas of the essay had rough transitions where the flow of ideas needs refinement. Both transitions and organization need attention.	Organization is evident; some transitions need work.	Both organization and transitions are solid.

Uniqueness

Content is commonplace and not particularly unique. This could be someone else's essay quite easily.	One or two elements are unique, but the remainder of the ideas are commonplace.	Essay contains mostly unique ideas. This could not easily be someone else's essay.	Essay is truly one of a kind, deeply personal, and original.

Comments:

actually read the answers. Do not recycle content from another essay that does not answer the question. Do not cut and paste an answer from elsewhere that is bland, overly general, or not applicable. Do not pivot and answer a question you would rather write about instead of the one we asked. We can tell when you do that.

The written elements of your application are a personal testimony and tell us why we should want to meet you in person. Again—the goal of the application is to get an interview. Schools typically interview only a tiny percentage of their applicant pools. At one of my schools we received about 15,000 applications and interviewed 725. At another school it was 288 interviews from 6,000 applications. If you make it into that interview phase, you are already receiving strong consideration for admission. If you do not maximize the writing in your application, it is akin to being asked in an interview if you would like to share something about yourself and answering "No, thank you." Seize the opportunity to write specific responses to each school and answer their questions thoroughly, passionately, and well. If you are having difficulty appealing to the school's mission in your responses, step back and ask yourself if you are a good fit for that school.

If you are going to cut and paste, please make sure you do not get sloppy. Every year I read essays for my school telling me how much an applicant wants to attend another school. True story. It's a dead giveaway that you did not spend much time on your supplemental, and it gives me wiggle room to not spend much time on your review. I figure you probably are not that interested in my school.

Advocate for Yourself

If you are interested in a school, you lose nothing by expressing that interest appropriately. It is very important to be your own advocate during the process. As I said before, we are managing the files of thousands of applicants; it is up to you to manage yours. It is acceptable to send an email expressing your interest, unless the school specifically asks you not to. If you have met someone from that school during a recruitment fair or event, reach out and send an email when your file is complete. Use your connections as much as possible to get noticed. It is a good idea to express continued interest through application updates and periodic emails, just don't overdo it. A general guideline would be one email after you have completed the supplemental (in the fall) and one email before interview season closes (in the winter) if you have not received an interview. If you interviewed and you have not heard back, you can follow up in March and again in April or May, depending on how your candidacy progresses. If there is an applicant portal, use that for updates and letters of interest. If the school has a portal for updates, that is likely the best way to ensure your updates are attached to your file. If you send emails they may have to be manually added by a staff member and may not be noted by a committee.

Alexis

Alexis was a candidate on our alternate list. She did well during the interview but had not initially received an offer. We were about six weeks from orientation and there had been little movement among our intended incoming class. My director received a call from Alexis asking if she could come in and meet with him. She showed up prepared with an update in hand. She was dressed as though it was a second interview, because it was. She spoke clearly and passionately about her desire to attend our school and also expressed that she understood it was a process and that things moving forward were uncertain. She discussed her plans to reapply and what she would be doing in the coming year to continue to prepare herself. She asked for feedback on her plans. We were impressed with Alexis. She presented herself professionally and confidently. She was assertive yet humble. When we had an unexpected withdrawal the following week, we made her an offer of admission.

Many schools do not work this way. Some schools have ranked alternate lists or different processes by which they extend offers. There are also many factors that impact admissions. That was a year for us that we had unique factors that ultimately resulted in a very small alternate list. I do not share this story to encourage you to show up at the schools you are considering and try to demand a meeting. You should not pepper a school with status calls or otherwise be obnoxious in promoting yourself. (I have some stories there, too—none with happy endings!) You absolutely must respect the boundaries of the admissions office and its personnel. Being a self-advocate means keeping your interest in the school and your file up to date at the schools where you are still seeking admission.

Letters of Intent

The closer a school is to its orientation date, the more it will take into consideration the stability of the incoming classes and ensuring that they are seated. The last thing schools want is movement on the class list a few days before school is going to start, because that means someone is finding out they are going to medical school with a few days' notice. Yes, applicants are elated no matter when they receive that acceptance phone call, but it is best to avoid last-minute shuffling. The later the season goes, the more likely offers will be extended to candidates with the greatest assurance of matriculation. Many schools pay attention to who has expressed continued interest and who may have sent letters of intent.

You should definitely tell your top school that they are your top choice, and this is essentially the purpose of a letter of intent. A letter of intent should only be sent to one school. If you try to tell everyone that they are your number one, it may backfire. (Plus there's that whole honesty and integrity thing, which is super important for future physicians.) If you are sending a letter, state why the school is your top choice. Hopefully these reasons are related to the school and your goals, not merely the location or some other triviality. If you want to submit the strongest possible letter of intent, state that you will withdraw from consideration at all other schools if given an offer (and of course be willing to follow through if you do so). This is especially important if you already have an acceptance at another school, but not your top choice. Again, professionalism applies here. Be truthful in your dealings with schools throughout the application process.

Follow the Rules

You can find the AAMC guidelines for what is expected of you in the Application and Acceptance Protocols for Applicants.[5] This is a set of agreed-on rules for all applicants that you will be held accountable for following. (There are similar rules that schools have agreed to abide by, which you can find in the AAMC Application and Acceptance Protocols for Admission Officers.[6]) The rules govern the earliest allowable offer date, the amount of money allowed for a deposit to hold your seat, and how long you can hold multiple offers. When you agree to use the AMCAS, you are agreeing to follow these rules. Make sure you know them so that you can demonstrate professionalism throughout the cycle. Knowing the protocols also ensures that your decision making is informed by the rules that schools must also follow.

Admissions Roulette

Many deans use some form of past data analysis to try and approximate who is likely to accept their offer and attend their school and how many total offers to make early in the cycle in order to land on the magic number of seats in the class. I get asked about this often when I do committee trainings: "How do you know how many offers to make to account for multiple offers but still get to the class target?" Welcome to the game of admissions roulette, my friends! I honestly lose a lot of sleep worrying about this every year. I do not want to oversubscribe the class and have too many students, but I also do not want to miss out on top candidates by waiting too long to make offers. The timing of offers matters because at some point applicants commit and begin transitioning their lives to prepare to attend their chosen school. If we make an offer too late, we may discover that we were the applicant's preferred school in April, but by June that may not be the case.

Applicants play a role in how the offers are timed. When applicants hold multiple seats, especially beyond deadlines, it causes chaos and uncertainty in admissions enrollment management. At the end of the cycle every applicant can only claim one seat. If you receive an offer for admission and you know you will not be attending that school, let the school know as soon as possible. There is another applicant waiting for news. Each year there are students who find out in June or July that they are accepted to medical school. This leaves very little time for them to transition their lives and prepare. Your behavior in the applicant universe affects others, so be a good citizen.

Complete Financial Aid Forms Early

Here is another important tip for the application season: Do your financial aid applications early. Always do your financial aid forms early at every school for which you remain in consideration. Sometimes when we are looking at late-season alternate lists we cross-check those lists against who has submitted financial aid information and when they submitted it. Our financial aid colleagues need to be able to package loans quickly, and if you have not sent in your forms, it causes a delay. Financial aid processes at schools vary, so pay attention and make sure you follow through with their requests so that you will receive consideration for all types of aid. If there is a deadline specified by financial aid, meet it. Know that I may also use your follow-through on financial aid to approximate your interest in my school. If you didn't bother to follow up on aid forms, are you really interested in attending? Or, if you were interested but failed to follow up, are your organizational skills up to par for medical school?

Transferring Is Rare

Here is another critical tip about choosing a medical school: no transferring. Choosing a medical school wisely is critical because that is going to be your home for the next four years. If you do not like it, you will have very few options.

Ibrahim

Ibrahim was accepted and came to our "second look" event. He was excited about being a part of the class and was in conversations with a few incoming students about getting an apartment together. In late June, he received an offer from his state school. Because it was less expensive and close to home and family, he felt pressured to go there. His parents wanted him close by, as he was the eldest of several children in a first-generation immigrant family. He called me before withdrawing and explained his decision. I was sad to lose him and wished him well.

Four months later I received a call from Ibrahim. He was not happy at his school. He said he was not struggling academically, just very unhappy and not receiving the support he needed. He asked me about transfer options—could he still come to my school? Could he get his seat back and start next year? I explained to him that he could not transfer schools like that—this was professional school, not undergrad. We do not allow you to port your offer to another year if you matriculate to another school. I offered encouragement and we talked about resources at his school that he could reach out to for support.

A few weeks later Ibrahim's father called me in distress. Ibrahim was considering withdrawing from his current school and reapplying the following year. I strongly advised against this option. When you apply through AMCAS there is a section for previous matriculation and it is associated with your ID number. All participating schools will know that you had a seat somewhere and did not complete that program. Many schools have admissions policies that keep them from considering applicants who had a seat somewhere and did not finish. I advised Ibrahim's father to help his son adjust and find resources to be successful and happy at his school. It would almost certainly end his career in medicine to withdraw and attempt to start over. This was a very painful lesson for Ibrahim and his family. You will be happy to know that he is doing well and was finally able to settle in and make the most of his experience.

Some medical schools occasionally allow transfers. Transfers are rare and only pending if there is space. The accreditation guidelines for medical schools provide guidelines for transfers and specifically limit transfers in the final year.[7] A very small number of students each year transfer between schools. Transfers from MD school to MD school usually happen between the second and third year, after a student has successfully completed the Step 1 licensing exam. Transfer applications typically consist of sending your previous AMCAS, current medical school transcripts, letters of recommendation, and an explanation as to why you are seeking a transfer. You will need to search each school individually to find out if the school accepts transfers or not, as there is no central clearinghouse.

Students must be in good standing to transfer. They cannot have performance issues, professionalism problems, or any liabilities per the accreditation rules. Remember when I said that admissions deans talk to each other? Well, student affairs deans do, too. They likely will have a phone conversation with each other about transfers prior to anything happening. They are colleagues in a very close knit professional network and want to act in the best interests of students and schools as a whole. A transfer student must have the endorsement of their home school in order to move to another school. The bottom line is: Choose your school wisely.

Choosing the Right Fit

Choose a medical school that meets your needs as a learner, suits your career goals, and offers the resources and opportunities you need to thrive. I realize that debt is a huge consideration these days, but I caution against choosing a school only for the lowest amount of loans. The goal of the entire ordeal is to reach your full potential in medicine. You must decide how much finances weigh in your overall goals and considerations. This is what you will be doing for the rest of your life and you owe it to yourself to thrive, not just survive. Reputation matters, loans matter, proximity to social support matters, but all these things will not make up for performance in school.

Cameron

Cameron was thirty-two years old when applying to medical school. Single and very independent, Cameron remodeled houses, always had projects happening, and was accustomed to working from home in the finance industry. Cameron was fortunate to have two offers for medical school—one from the state school and one from a private school that was perceived to be more prestigious. The private school also offered a half tuition scholarship, which made it slightly less money than the state school. Cameron was drawn to the reputation and prestige of the private school as a perceived career asset. The fact that it would be slightly less in loans was also appealing. Cameron and I spoke about the decision. Cameron chose to sell a home, move, and attend the private school several states away.

The school chosen had a small student body, and Cameron struggled to fit in. Everyone was younger and still into partying pretty hard. Cameron got along with people but was not accustomed to having an entire peer group of another age and felt out of place. The school was remote, so Cameron did not have other outlets that might be available in a larger city. The school also required lecture attendance from 8 a.m. to 5 p.m. five days a week. Cameron did not learn best in lecture. Having completed an MBA through an executive program and accustomed to having autonomy, Cameron liked when there was a lot of independent learning and studying and was not used to having to be in a classroom so many hours a day.

Cameron spent evenings from six to midnight studying but fell behind and began to struggle on exams. There wasn't enough time to study the way that Cameron needed to learn best. Cameron tried to adapt, but the pace of the courses was too demanding. Feeling underprepared and incredibly stressed, Cameron tried to delay the Step 1 exam but couldn't. Ultimately, Cameron underperformed in medical school and on Step 1 and ended up changing specialty and professional direction. Eventually Cameron recovered, graduated, and matched into residency, but with options that were more limited than originally imagined at the beginning of the journey.

If Cameron had looked beyond the scholarship offer and prestige and spent more time exploring fit, this story might have turned out differently. This student might have avoided the performance stress experienced during medical school. This is why I say that you cannot choose a school based on money or perceived prestige. The experience of those four years matters personally and professionally. The better the fit the more you will be able to thrive and actually enjoy medical school. What is the educational environment like? Are there small groups? Lectures? Hands-on learning? Will the learning environment meet your specific needs? Do your homework and investigate all these important issues. Inventory what you think you need to be successful and look for a school that has those resources.

Manage Your Candidacy

Another important aspect of the application process is ensuring that you actively maintain your candidacy at schools you wish to attend. If you decide you do not wish to attend a school, withdraw your application. It is up to you to decide whether a seat at a school that is not ideal for you is better than no seat at all. It is rare that applicants interview and withdraw before a decision is made, but it happens. Perhaps they have an offer elsewhere or have another reason for withdrawing—we do not take it personally. Admissions deans appreciate your being prompt and decisive about your candidacy. It helps us manage our processes and allows us to get our classes seated efficiently. I do not advise that you turn down a seat in the current cycle to apply to a different school the following cycle. Given how arduous and expensive the process is and the overall odds of getting a seat, there is no guarantee of another offer. Occasionally students have good reasons for receiving offers and not matriculating or deferring, but wanting to go to another school that you perceive is better is not one of them. If you do your homework in the first place, the odds are highly unlikely anyway. If you have a geographic restriction or other considerations that limit where you can attend, apply within those parameters.

9

Understand the Graduate/ Professional School Context

Dear Dean Nakae,

I'm very frustrated. I've applied to medical school twice and have not been successful. I have a 3.69 GPA. My MCAT [Medical College Admission Test] score is 514 and I only took the test once. I have strong extracurricular activities and leadership, plus my research is being published next month. All my letter writers have told me that they wrote me strong letters. One is even from the chair of Molecular Biology that I have worked with for three years. I volunteer all the time since I've had to take a gap year to apply again. I had a few interviews my first cycle but did not get any offers. This time I did not receive any interview offers. I'm disappointed and wondering what to do next. I'm also frustrated at the process because my friends with lower grades and MCATs got in these past two cycles and I didn't. I don't think it's fair. I don't understand what I am doing wrong. Honestly, I feel like I've been unfairly discriminated against in this process. What do you recommend?

Sincerely,

Frustrated Applicant

Before I reply to messages such as this one I try to step back and assess what I see every day from my vantage point as an admissions dean that applicants cannot see. I realize their perspective is different and they may have incomplete information. Where is the disconnect in this applicant's experiences and his assessment of what's going on? What is happening at the micro, mezzo, and macro levels that has yielded these outcomes? Is this an issue of inaccurate self-appraisal? Poor application strategy? Poor people skills? What kind of feedback does this applicant need to move forward?

Medical School Admissions by the Numbers

Let's first tackle the macro-level: graduate and professional school admissions. The medical education data publicly available from the Association of American Medical Colleges (AAMC) is a starting point.[1] The website aamc.org/data has charts detailing information on applicants and matriculants. For the 2018–2019 cycle there were 52,777 applicants for 21,622 seats.[2] That means 41 percent of the applicants had a seat at the end of the cycle, and 59 percent (31,155 applicants) did not. The average grade point average (GPA) for those applicants was 3.57. The average GPA for those that subsequently matriculated was 3.72. The average MCAT score for applicants was 505.6, with a standard deviation of 9.3, and the average score for those who matriculated was 511.2, with a standard deviation of 6.5. What these numbers tell you is that there are thousands of applicants, presumably with solid to excellent academic preparation, who were not offered seats. The differences in numbers are not enough to determine who will receive a spot and who will not. Furthermore, schools across the country use far more than numbers to evaluate a candidate.

Public data from the AAMC reveals the overall acceptance rate for applicants and matriculants by combinations of MCAT scores and GPAs.[3] According to the data, applicants with GPAs greater than 3.79 were accepted 66.3 percent of the time regardless of MCAT score. For those in the next GPA tier of 3.6 to 3.79, the acceptance rate was 47.9 percent. Another way to say this is that 33.7 percent of the students who applied to medical school with

GPAs of 3.79 and above were *not* accepted. For applicants with MCAT scores of 514 to 517, the acceptance rate was 73.8 percent regardless of GPA. Even for MCATs of 517 and above (very high scores) the acceptance rate was 83.7 percent. Are these higher than the overall acceptance rate? Yes! But they are not 100 percent. Even when you look at a near-perfect to perfect GPA (3.79 and above) *and* a super-high MCAT score (517+), there are still 11.2 percent of applicants who did not receive any acceptances. For the next tier, students with a GPA of 3.6 to 3.79 and an MCAT score of 514 to 517 (the tier that our frustrated applicant is in), the data indicates that 25 percent of candidates with those credentials did not receive *any* offers. Did every allopathic school in the United States and Puerto Rico say no to all those applicants with amazing numbers? Yes. Getting in is about more than numbers.

Planning for All Possible Outcomes

Allopathic medicine is competitive, and that's an understatement. The bottom line is there are thousands of qualified candidates who will not have a seat at the end of each cycle. More than half of them will have to reapply. Having strong numbers is not the determining factor in whether a student will earn one of those 21,622 seats. Candidates who go into the process believing that there is no other outcome than to get a seat will be the most disappointed and most unprepared if they find themselves having to reapply. If you were planning a road trip and you knew in advance that one of the roads would be closed, but you weren't sure which one until you got to the intersection, wouldn't you plan accordingly? If the weather app on your phone said 60 percent chance of rain, would you pack an umbrella?

Savvy applicants accept this alternate-route reality and are resilient when facing rejection. Humble applicants who acknowledge that the process is competitive and that there are thousands of phenomenal candidates in the pool will fare better in the long run. The application cycle is a year, so it is wise to plan accordingly and to pursue multiple options simultaneously based on all possible outcomes so that you can continue the course if you are not successful getting a seat the first, second, or third time around. I promise you that as a dean, I am well aware that I miss talent every year. It is very difficult to go from 15,000 applications to 165 students or from 6,000 applications to 75 students. The process is not perfect. If you love medicine, plan accordingly and do not be afraid to try again. You will be in good company.

Now that we have addressed the numbers, let's talk about the fact that admission to medical school (and all graduate and professional schools) is far different from the undergraduate admission process. Whereas at the undergrad level there are enough seats for everyone to go somewhere, this is not the case at the graduate level. The world is full of happy people who at some point wanted to go to dental school, pharmacy school, business school, and so on. If things did not go according to plan, they regrouped, figured out another career option, and went for that. They accepted the variability in possible outcomes and found ways to use their gifts to benefit the world and earn a living. These days I see too many applicants who accuse the entire system of being wrong if they do not get their way. Rather than accept the odds, they believe everyone is wrong for not giving them what they sought.

A Seat in the Profession

Similarly, unlike the general nature of undergraduate education, a professional or graduate-level education carries far more weight. Admissions personnel are offering you a seat *in the profession*, which is not the same thing as a seat *in the classroom*. Physicians who are ultimately deciding if they want that person as a future colleague are the ones evaluating applicants. In an undergraduate setting, the enrollment management is broad and the admissions officers are professionals who carefully select students to enroll. Depending on the size of the school, the admissions personnel may never meet or see the students they select. In medical school, the individuals selecting you will be seated next to you in classrooms, teaching you in small groups, rounding with you in the hospital, and taking direct responsibility for your career success and graduation. In undergraduate admissions you have to be the right fit for the institution writ large; in medical school admissions you have to be the right fit for the specific people who will be charged with your education. In other words, if something goes wrong, you will be their problem. This is how deans and faculty view the process. We are going to be *personally* responsible for you. You will be our future colleague and you will carry the name of our institution forever.

Every medical school requires an interview as part of the admissions process. You must not only appear well prepared and well rounded on paper, you also must possess strong interpersonal skills and social skills. We have already shown how, according to the data, each year thousands of candidates with very high grades and test scores do not get a seat at any school. It is likely they received interviews and were not made offers. This is strong evidence that medical schools across the board look for far more than numeric characteristics in choosing their next class of physicians.

Enrollment Management Factors

At the mezzo level are all the factors involved in the various admissions processes at schools across the country. The timing of applications matters. The smaller details matter: Classification of letters of recommendation, premed coursework, and credit hours in specific classes might make a difference in one person's candidacy over another. Deadlines, answers to supplemental applications, and state residency can all influence an application's outcome as it makes its way through each school's unique process.

Many of these factors are within an applicant's control, but some of them are not. The world of admissions enrollment management is vast, and there are many considerations that go into selecting and shaping a class. Each school occupies a position in the marketplace of schools competing for students. Therefore schools are looking for students who are both a good fit for what they are offering and are also likely to attend if offered a seat. Some of the factors are not related to you personally; they are larger issues that combine to create the demographic makeup of the class (e.g., men/women, public/private schools, state residencies, language skills).

Mission Matters

Not to be overlooked, every school has a mission, and that mission dictates the weight the school places on certain experiences or applicant characteristics. Think of this as the equivalent of the way we use personality traits in the dating world. For example, school A may frown on community college work, while school B is neutral. School A may be seeking students with significant basic science research, while school B may be looking for students interested in studying public health. Sometimes it's not personal. Before you apply you should spend time on the school websites learning more about each school's mission and choosing schools to which you are well suited. Students must use caution against viewing rejections as personal assaults on their character and qualifications. The truth is, you may not have been the right fit for the school, or something about the timing of your application caused you to miss out.

If the school has a primary care focus and your application strengths were mainly in research and innovation, why would the school choose you? If the school's mission is to serve underserved communities and your application discussed entrepreneurship and your desire to earn an MBA as well, do you think you would be able to thrive at that school? Applicants should not apply to a school without considering the specific mission of the school and how their experiences, passions and preparations stack up. I often hear applicants say they just want to get in anywhere and it doesn't matter where they go. The irony is that when applicants apply with a scattershot strategy without regard to mission, it means that schools have to wade through more applications and ultimately have less time to read each one.

If you are the best cancer biology researcher in the world and you apply to a doctoral program that specializes in genomics, the admissions committee may not select you. It won't be because you aren't smart, capable, and accomplished in your field; it will be because they do not want to squelch your potential by taking you away from a program where you could truly thrive and make a significant contribution to cancer biology. They also would recognize that they do not have the faculty expertise to develop your talent and to maximize your contribution to the program while in it. If there are no faculty to teach and mentor you in that area, it kind of defeats the purpose of what you are seeking—an education. It is actually out of respect for your potential that the program did not choose you. The focus and mission of the school matters. Your expressed interests and goals matter.

Finding Meaning in Rejection

Now for the micro level. This is always the difficult gut check that applicants have to face if rejected. Sometimes when an admissions committee says no they are saying "not yet." We often discuss the trajectory of development for candidates and feel they would benefit from more time preparing or maturing before they take a seat in our class. Other times when we say no we mean "no for us." This means we feel we do not have the environment you may need to thrive and we think you would be a better fit somewhere else. And yes, occasionally when we say no we mean "hell no," but that is actually more rare than you would think.

Applicants who are contemplating trying again have to confront the tough questions: What kind of person are you? How do you behave when you don't get what you want? What can you improve on or do differently next time? Getting into medical school is less about the accolades on your application and has everything to do with the authentic person that you are. You cannot fake altruism, empathy, or genuineness. So, while you may have stacked your resume for college admissions with activities and awards a few years ago, that strategy simply won't work with medical school. Everyone applying to medical school went to college, therefore they are *all* trying that same thing. Now for some straight talk that may be difficult to hear.

Dear Frustrated Applicant,

You have asserted in your correspondence to me that you believe yourself more deserving of admission than your friends. This should give you pause. Are you the kind of friend you wish to have? What would your friends think if they knew you felt this way? On what grounds have you assessed yourself to be better? At my school, I wish to have students who cheer for each other's successes, not sulk in resentment at their own failures. A friend's triumph should not be your loss. If you cannot find a way to be disappointed without externalizing that on your friends, I need you to think about that.

You have also asserted, by insinuating that you are a better applicant than your friends, that you believe our admissions system is somehow flawed and that you know more than my admissions committee. This is also of great concern. We have read more than 10,000 applications this year alone, how many have you read? We decide what factors we use in selecting our students, and for you to assert that they are wrong because they did not yield you a spot is, quite frankly, arrogant and concerning.

This is a crossroads moment where you get to decide whether you take full and complete responsibility for yourself and therefore control your future, or whether you allow your shame and disappointment to distract you toward fear and self-pity. You will need to ask yourself these questions: Do I deeply know why I want to be a physician? Have I actively interrogated this goal? What personal values underscore this desire? How have I shown these values in my pursuit of this goal? What am I willing to sacrifice in pursuit of this goal? If I don't get what I am ultimately after, what's my plan to move forward? Is this goal about making a difference in the world, or it is about making a difference only with the MD that I believe I am entitled to, no matter what?

The first hallmark of character is how we behave when no one is watching or keeping score. The second hallmark is how we behave when we do not get what we want. The third hallmark of character is what we are willing to do for others. It may be time to start working on the character section of your application. The good news is you are probably not alone. There are likely more than 30,000 applicants who may be facing the exact same challenge.

Lovingly,
Dean Nakae

10

Professionalism and People Skills in a Digital Era

I like to tell this funny story about a neighbor's child who used to come over to our house all the time with tablet in hand. My partner and I encourage our children to play outside, interact with people, and be creative and curious. This child would come over and ask for our Wi-Fi password without even making eye contact. One beautiful Chicago day the neighbor's child appeared in the living room while the rest of the kids were outside riding bikes and, staring blankly at the tablet screen, asked for the Wi-Fi password. My partner said, "Sure. You ready? It's g-e-t-o-u-t-s-i-d-e." The child looked up and said, "It didn't work." My partner laughed, "Oh yes it did."

There is no substitute for human interaction. The way to build people skills is to *interact with people*. More specifically, learn to build skills with people that you meet for the first time or with whom you might not otherwise interact. This is what you will be doing every single day as a doctor. It's a big deal. If you cannot connect with a patient effectively you will not be able to do your job. Even if you are the most knowledgeable person on the science of medicine, without an accurate and complete patient history you cannot be effective. Without patient trust, things have the potential to go wrong. When we interview you, we need to see your confident, warm, effective people skills. We are assessing whether you can successfully communicate and connect with us during a brief interview. When we meet you at recruitment fairs or internship interviews, we are assessing your people skills. If you feel you are weak in this area, you will need to reread chapter 7 (The Secret to a Competitive Edge) about the growth zone.

Connection Mindset

I was at a recruitment fair a few years ago and a student sauntered up to the table. He was wearing flip-flops, half a shirt, and a hat turned backward. He didn't make any eye contact with me and casually thumbed through the brochures. He then said, "Like, what kind of school is this? What's the deal with your school? Like, is it a chill school or super competitive? I mean like, how do you all, like, look at people from California?"

I then introduced myself as the admissions dean, much to his surprise. While this was not a medical school interview, it was a recruitment fair. I am there to meet prospective students and to identify talent for my school. I am not saying he should have worn a suit, but it was evident that he gave no forethought to his attire or how he would present himself. A recruitment fair is a pre-professional venue, like a dress rehearsal for entering the profession. The student should have prepared to ask specific questions related to his goals in medicine. He should have composed himself better so that he would be memorable in a positive way. The student should have attended with a connection mindset, not a consumer one. A consumer mindset says, "What am I getting out of this?" Your primary intention is to *take*. You walk around, grab the free stuff, and seek information. A connection mindset says, "Who can I meet? What can I learn?" Your primary intention is to *interact*. When you intentionally make connections and ask thoughtful questions you build relationships by presenting your authentic self.

Professional Writing

Speaking of presenting yourself, please capitalize, spell correctly, and use proper grammar. Always. In all aspects of your application, for all correspondence with everything to do with your professional life, you must attend to proper grammar. No exceptions. Different generations are reading your file, and not everyone appreciates hashtags as much as you do. (In fact, most of us call those pound signs.) And no creative liberties, either. Do not try to format the page so it looks like a river or a cross. Do not write an allegory that makes no sense for a personal statement. Do not use texting phrases like "LOL" or "TL;DR" in your professional writing. Do not put links to your Etsy crochet gallery or your YouTube channel. Allow yourself no creative liberties that are over the top or outside the norm. Your application is not the place for that. Trust me, it will not translate well and it will not be perceived the way you intend.

Application Photos

Professionalism in a digital era can be challenging. The photos you share on social media and the photos you submit for your application should *not* be one and the same. No red solo cups, please. No nondescript children of color standing beside you. No photos on boats, mountains, camels, or roller-coasters. No hats, sports jerseys, scrubs, or masquerade gear. No photos cropped from a wedding line. No third-grade throwbacks. No black-and-white artistry or Snapchat filters. No creative paintings. No car selfies. Just take a nice professional photo like the one you would see in a physician provider profile. And please smile. We do not wish to see your grumpy expression or a painful look on your face. While your passport photo may be an easy and tempting option, don't use it because you are not allowed to smile in passport photos. We like happy students! Please pay attention to the upload instructions so that your photo is not super tiny or sideways. (As a side note: Your photo might also become your student ID on the first day of school. I had a former student years ago who sent in his football photo because it was one he had easily on hand. That photo was used for his school ID and for the class photo roster. His friends and family teased him endlessly about it.)

I should take a moment to explain that some schools use photos in the process so that we can remember applicants and distinguish them during discussion or subsequent recruitment events. But as the saying goes, "A picture is worth a thousand words." We often wonder what applicants are thinking when they submit inappropriate or lazy photos for their professional medical school applications.

Character Counts

Your behavior is indicative of your character. Professionalism is essentially the development of your character in your professional and personal roles over time. We take character very seriously. There was a rule in one of my admissions offices that we named after an applicant who drove us crazy. He continually harassed my staff calling nearly every day. We keep track of calls, emails, portal visits, and inquiries. We want to know how much you are interacting with us. This student logged over fifty phone calls after his interview. He demonstrated impatience, selfishness, poor impulse control, entitlement, and poor empathy by calling us so much.

Schools receive thousands of applications—if everyone called that much we would never get anything done. Although the applicant had managed to impress both interviewers, the committee was made aware of his behavior. Remember that discussion about fit? Remember how I said committee members and decision makers will be directly involved in your education? Well, committee members imagined themselves having to deal with a student like that for four years. They all voted no, and it was unanimous.

There are little things within your application that send messages about who you are and how you conduct yourself. Readers extrapolate all sorts of qualities and characteristics from your application. We try to square these impressions with your performance in the classroom, on exams, and in testimonials from letters of recommendation. If your email is hemptoker@ . . . or armcandy@ . . . for your professional school application, we question your judgment. (Apologies if these are actual email addresses of real people—I just made them up.) We wonder if you are giving a professional school application the weight and attention it deserves. We question your maturity. Do not crack jokes or allow any element of your application and professional profile to be remotely inappropriate or immature. We look at everything. Everything.

Social Media

Many schools have policies not to seek additional information about candidates on social media, but that is not a reason to act out online. The words you post should not be different from those you would speak to someone face-to-face. The memes you post should not be different from those you would hang in your house or carry through the streets publicly. Your professional reputation is established in the history you leave of your behavior online and elsewhere. Be thoughtful and use good judgment. Once you are a student you will be held accountable for all behaviors online and in person. Learn to temper your reactions and engage respectfully.

People Skills

Developing confident interpersonal skills takes time and practice. Eye contact, body language, posture, gesture—these things take years to master. In order to relate to others effectively you need to be confident in yourself and your ability to interact. Nothing sharpens those skills like a customer service job or a volunteer gig that pushes you to interact more.

Perry

Perry had been working and living on his own since he was sixteen years old. He was the only person in his family with a bank account, a car, and a high school diploma, let alone a college degree. He waited tables and put himself through undergrad. During summers he worked two jobs, one as a waiter and one as a lifeguard and server at a country club. I was curious as to how he got the job and what he had learned working in a very different environment. (I am completely unfamiliar with country club cultures and lifestyles as well.) He laughed when I asked him to explain the hidden rules of the club, but he knew what I meant. His answer fascinated me.

> Working there I learned that people really operate by the same rules no matter where they are from. They want their expectations met, and if those expectations aren't met, they want to be heard. It sounds really simple, but that's it. The club's expectations are that life is easier there than at home. All the amenities the club offers are things that people expect. They want hot food, clean towels, clean tables, friendly staff that are willing to help, etc. When those expected norms are violated, then they want to air their grievances and feel validated. The larger the violation, the more power the person hearing them has to have.
>
> I learned to deal with difficult situations. I learned to handle conflict graciously and effectively between patrons and fellow employees. I learned to step back and not take things personally. By removing myself and thinking of things more objectively, I could think more clearly and stay focused on finding a solution. When things are heated that's when people lose their heads and get upset. This never works. It doesn't help any situation to be upset or emotional.

Not only is Perry a good communicator, he is confident. He has dealt with conflict in difficult situations that helped him strengthen his skills. He is at ease speaking with almost anyone and it shows. His bandwidth for effective communication is strong.

Professionalism Guidelines

Professionalism has been a hot topic in medical education for many years now. We know that students who do not display professionalism grow up to be physicians with professionalism and licensing board disciplinary issues.[1] Previous generations constantly lament that the younger generations have no idea how to be professional or what that even means. Older folk frequently express frustration that younger people have to be told every single thing. So here is my quick and simple guide to professionalism for aspiring medical students and beyond.

1. Be on time. Pretty simple. It says a great deal about your level of investment and how much you care. If you will not be on time, let others know. Take responsibility for your actions.

2. Respect others' time. Every admissions season we have candidates cancel interviews at the last minute and we are unable to fill their spot. Often they live hundreds of miles away and it was obvious that they knew many days before that they wouldn't be coming to interview. Worse, sometimes people are complete no-shows. There are medical students making arrangements during study time to read your file and interview you. There are doctors rearranging clinic hours to interview you. Be respectful. This is not like a tour bus ticket you decided not to use. If you cannot honor a commitment, let people know.

3. Meet your deadlines. Working with students day in and day out, I find it astonishing how many students do not understand what a deadline means. Do not call my admissions office and ask for an extension on your AMCAS on November 2 when the deadline is November 1. The application window is several months. There are literally *no* valid excuses or reasons why you should not be able to make your application on time. Furthermore, when you become a student and then a physician, the deadline rule is even more important. If I ask you to complete immunization requirements by a certain date, there's a reason. If you do not do that, you won't be able to go to clinic. Period. If you anticipate having difficulty with a deadline, let people know well beforehand. Be a problem solver.

4. Follow the rules. When it comes to guidelines and rules, don't be that person who thinks you are special and you don't have to follow rules. If you genuinely need an exception, ask respectfully and in a way that fully acknowledges you are not entitled to one.

Do not look for technical loopholes in rules to get away with things you know the rules are intended to prohibit. Yes, you may prevail in the immediate term on a technicality, but it does not speak well of your character to exploit a loophole.

5. Manage your priorities and understand that not everyone may share them. Your best friend's bachelorette party on the same day as an exam is not my problem, it's yours. It is therefore your job to resolve this conflict according to your priorities. While the choice is yours to make, you cannot control the consequences. Understand that as you become an adult you will increasingly wish to be in two or more places at once. You will wish there were more than twenty-four hours in a day or that you did not have to sleep. (Trust me, I wish this daily.) Do not allow your personal life to spin out of control and expect others to pick up the pieces when things do not go well. Your social life, travel excursions, and shopping habits will probably need to be altered in pursuit of your long-term goals. The older I get the more I am torn between the multiple demands on my time. I am constantly choosing between equally good things, not between good and bad. Learn to prioritize now.

6. Use respectful speech. In email, in person, and on social media, your words are a reflection of who you are. You are what you post. Use titles and salutations in your correspondence with individuals who have formal authority. Treat everyone with respect, from the administrative assistant to the dean to the custodian working on the grounds outside the school. My committee once denied admission to a candidate we all supported because he swore during his interview and it was noted as a professionalism concern. Even though he had many faculty members who valued his candidacy, in the end, no one could deny that being on one's best behavior includes not swearing.

7. Accept feedback and implement it. The people who really care about you are the ones who tell you that you have a booger hanging out of your nose. The people who care will tell you, not let you continue without being told that you're doing something wrong or contrary to your goals. Throughout my career I have

constantly sought feedback on how I could improve and what I should be doing better. Although at some points when I fell short the feedback was hard to hear, I took it to heart and used it to continue my path forward. If you are going to ask for feedback, implement it and grow from it. Do something with the feedback you receive.

8. Learn to manage conflict. This is perhaps one of the most difficult aspects of professionalism, even for many seasoned professionals. When there is disagreement and discord, learn to be communicative, to remain solution focused, and to keep things confidential. Do not gossip to several people about a problem. Take time to address the matter with the source. Careers are marathons, not sprints, and often the people you disagree with in year two of your career are the ones you'll be collaborating with a few years later. Disagree without being disagreeable. Do not speak ill of others. People will respect your integrity and will want you on their team.

Professionalism is also good judgment about how to present yourself or approach a situation. What picture should you submit? What is the dress code? Should you directly approach someone or go through their assistant? These are all a matter of judgment. If you aren't sure, find someone you trust to ask. Don't assume your behavior is always going to be the norm.

Professionalism is being engaged and representing yourself well during interactions. I had an applicant a few years ago who was unsuccessful gaining admission twice. I received several faculty and friend pleas for this applicant, including an in-person visit from his father (see the chapter 11 for my advice for parents and friends if you want to know my thoughts on that). By the way, I cannot discuss your application with your parents. It's not allowed, so parent meetings are inherently awkward and unproductive. The applicant had not taken us up on the advice to meet with admissions for feedback between application one and application two. After application two, he reluctantly met with me.

The first thing I noticed was that he looked very different in his admissions photo than in person. When I asked about it, he said he was self-conscious about his acne and preferred the old photo. The photo he submitted would not have been my top choice; he was not smiling in the photo and had a slightly awkward expression on his face, and it was obviously outdated. (Remember what I said about photos!) We discussed his application and I got the sense that he was meeting with me as a formality, not because he really wanted feedback. The most impressive aspect of the candidate's file was his research, which he had done with faculty connected to his physician parent. He had very little service and community engagement compared to applicants typically considered for interview at my school. I advised, based on his previous interview reports and application components, that he work on people skills, find some community endeavors he wished to impact, and challenge himself interpersonally in the coming year.

Fast-forward two admissions cycles and his application came across my desk again. More faculty pleas and advocacy for his candidacy filled my voicemail and email. He came to my office to meet with me in the middle of the current admissions cycle. We discussed his preparation since our last meeting. He said he was doing a master's program in another state. I asked about service endeavors and community engagement, referring to the previous advice I gave. He replied that he did not have time to do service because the academic demands of his master's program were too steep.

This applicant wasted my time twice. It is maddening to dedicate time to someone who has no desire to listen or take advice. Why would I encourage my committee to consider someone who has engaged with me in this way? What behaviors might we expect from this person if he were to become one of our students? His academic credentials were solid and he had no need for additional science coursework or a higher Medical College Admission Test (MCAT) score. His people skills needed work and in our second meeting he demonstrated that quite clearly.

Your actions communicate more to decision makers than you may intend. At one of my schools, each interview day began with a group information session promptly at 9:00 A.M. The director ran the session and usually spent an hour meeting the candidates and presenting information about the school. One interview morning I was rushing to a 9:15 meeting. I came up the stairwell, which was outside our office door, and I saw a candidate talking on his phone. It was 9:13. I'm not sure if he knew I was the dean, but just then he hurriedly hung up and walked into the information session—late.

I have no idea what was happening in the candidate's life that necessitated his being on his phone during a medical school interview. Yes, you heard me, an interview. *The entire day is your interview.* Every moment you are with us you are being evaluated and assessed. I specifically asked the director if the candidate had mentioned anything about an emergency or if he had later apologized for being late to the group information session. He had not communicated any extenuating circumstances that day, nor did he contact any of us after the session. Being on your phone when you are supposed to be engaged with other humans is poor professional behavior. It communicates to us that your medical school admission is not a priority to you, or it may indicate poor impulse control. Being on your phone says that you would rather do something else than engage with us about your candidacy.

We assume that when you come for an interview you are on the best behavior you know how to exhibit, so when we see these lapses in professionalism, they concern us. We wonder if you will have the self-control and maturity to put away your phone during mandatory meetings, trainings, patient encounters, or important lectures. We wonder if you have not yet figured out that you cannot be in two places at once and that your performance will suffer because your interpersonal judgment is poor. On the one hand you might think, "Wow, that's harsh. He was only ten minutes late. Maybe he had a good reason to be on his phone." I do not disagree. All I know is there were more than 600 candidates who interviewed at my school that season that were on time and were not taking hallway calls during planned activities.

Honesty

Professionalism also means demonstrating maturity. We view applicants who lack the ability to self-regulate as red flags. Once an applicant told us on interview day that he had been obligated to pay a $1,000 deposit at another medical school to hold his seat. This is against the rules for allopathic schools participating in the American Medical College Application Service (AMCAS), or the common application service. My director was concerned and relayed this information to me. Later that afternoon I called the admissions dean at the school in question. She was a colleague of mine but relatively new in her role. I explained what the applicant had reported and she confirmed it was false. She even sent me a screenshot of the fee page for her school. Why would this applicant lie to us about something like this? It was unnecessary and foolish. Perhaps he was exaggerating, maybe he was mistaken and not paying attention to what the deposit actually was. Either way, those are poor characteristics of a future doctor. Bottom line: Professionalism applies to everyone everywhere!

PART IV

Support Team Advice

11

Advice for Parents and Friends

Parental involvement in the college education of children has never been higher.[1] At the undergraduate college level, parents are part of the process more than ever before. This is somewhat normative, as freshman students are exiting high school and transitioning to a college environment—perhaps living on their own for the first time. In graduate and professional education we deal exclusively with what we expect to be fully independent adults. We assume that candidates are independent because they are achieving in college and seeking career entry. Many medical schools have programming for parents and families *after* candidates are admitted. If I am being honest, parental involvement in the admissions process is a royal pain for me every year. I share my perspective as a dean to help both applicants and parents understand where the boundaries should be and why.

We host open house information sessions during our season as a way for applicants to learn more about our institution and meet our current students. These are casual events meant to showcase our school and provide an open forum for prospective students to ask questions. That's how it should work.

Evelyn

Evelyn showed up for an open house one bright spring day. She was eager, with her notebook and pen in hand. She was at the front of the line for check-in first thing in the morning. She had not registered in advance, mainly because she was not a prospective student. She was here with her son, Caleb, a premed student. As they stepped up to the check-in desk, Evelyn dominated the interaction and gave their names. Evelyn made small talk about where they were from and how they had heard about our school. Evelyn reached out to grab the folder of materials and ushered Caleb to a seat in the front that she had chosen. Throughout the session Evelyn participated in a lively manner, asking questions and enjoying the perspectives that the current students shared. Caleb was attentive but didn't say much. By the end of the day it was clear to us who wanted to go to medical school. Maybe we would see an application from Evelyn soon?

Unfortunately, this type of scenario is not uncommon. We see parents overstepping all the time and doing things for their precious children that they simply should not do. I have seen parents attending recruitment fairs for their kids, collecting information, and handing representatives their child's business card and resume. If your child is admitted to medical school you will not attend lectures or small groups with them. You will not write papers, evaluate standardized patients, or take exams. Your child will be on their own.

Part of our assessment of someone's ability to thrive in medical school is based on their independence, coping skills, life skills, and communication skills. If you eclipse your child by hovering and meddling, we will not be able to assess these skills and will likely assume they are lacking. We often ask ourselves if students are truly motivated or if they are simply applying to medical school because of their parents. Those of us on the other side have seen students walk away from medicine, citing as the reason, "I never wanted this anyway; it was all because of my parents."

If your child is a strong candidate, they will not need your help getting into medical school. I repeat, if your child is a strong candidate, they will not need your help! You have to trust that you have taught them well and that their character, experiences, and preparation are excellent. You have to be confident that their ability to learn about a program and make a successful application to that program is intact. If you doubt any of these areas, you should not proceed by trying to run interference through admissions. If you are feeling insecure about your child's odds of acceptance, consider speaking with your child to express your concerns. This is your child's journey and there may be some aspects they simply have to learn on their own. Consider helping your child do a self-assessment and create a plan to improve in areas you both identify. In the end, every student needs organic confidence that they achieved their seat in the class and they deserve to be there. Your meddling could potentially take that away.

We do not like receiving emails or phone calls from parents about our requirements, policies, or practices. We wonder why the applicant is not asking these questions on their own. We question the applicant's motivation if they aren't leading the way. A few years ago my team noted that an applicant's mother had come to interview day with her. During the transitions between tours, lunch, and information sessions, the team met the applicant's mother. We were confused as to why the mother sat right outside our office all day. My team even asked her if she needed anything a few times because it was more than awkward! Later in the cycle, when comprising our alternate list, the uncertainty of the mother's involvement/presence came up as a possible concern. We were unsure about the boundaries and the independence of the candidate. We were not able to resolve this concern and ultimately did not prioritize the candidate. There may have been a good reason for the situation, but we will never know. No one else brought a parent to interview day.

Furthermore, going through the admissions process once and being successful does not make someone an expert any more than surviving cancer makes someone an oncologist. Some physician parents feel that because they were accepted into medical school years ago they are equipped to advise their child. While a parent's advice can be helpful and encouraging, it isn't always. Much has changed over the years when it comes to medical school application and enrollment. A parent's advice is given through their biased lens of what they know about their child; it may also be outdated, impractical, or incorrect.

The more we hear from you as a parent and not your child, who is the student applying, the more concerned we grow about the student's motivation and ability to thrive independently. If you have tried speaking with your child and it hasn't worked, maybe they need to go through the process and experience the outcomes in order to learn and grow. As a parent you can be a great backup singer, just never the lead. This is not your show, nor your career journey.

While writing emails to the dean may ease your anxiety or make you feel as though you are helping, it does not sway the votes of committee members. It stands to reason that parents cannot be objective about their own children. We all think our kids are great and that they deserve the success. We want what is best for them and we want their dreams to come true, especially if we know they have worked hard. Exercise some restraint and give your child space. In all my years in medical education I have never had an applicant that was happy that their parents contacted me. They are usually embarrassed, apologetic, horrified, or shocked. There has never been an instance where the committee has been grateful for parental involvement because it added something important to an applicant's candidacy that we could not get elsewhere.

Be aware that if you or another family member writes a letter of recommendation for your child we often do not give it much weight. In fact, we wonder why those students cannot get letters outside their family. If a relative writes a letter of recommendation for an applicant and does not disclose their relationship in the letter it can be damaging. If the relationship becomes known to the committee it appears duplicitous. If you are an alum or faculty member and you wish to recommend your child, inquire of the school through the proper/preferred channels—usually the alumni affairs or development office. Alumni affairs may have a formal communication channel with admissions to ensure that applicants related or associated with alums are not overlooked. Note that this policy varies greatly by school.

Because of privacy guidelines, we cannot share information with a parent about their child's candidacy. We cannot share any candidate's information with anyone other than the candidate without their authorization. Realize that as a parent you may be misinformed or underinformed about the situation. Every year we get calls from parents asking about their child's application and our records show the person never applied or never completed the supplemental application, but we cannot share anything. One season I received an angry letter from a parent whose son was not accepted that lauded the character and goodness of his son. What the applicant's father did not know was that his son had several institutional actions for problematic behavior during his undergraduate years. The American Medical College Application Service (AMCAS) requires that applicants disclose these citations. It was a heartbreaking situation for my staff to witness the disconnect and be unable to offer an explanation to the father.

How to Be a Supportive Parent

Now that I have provided my perspective on well-meaning parents and their involvement in a child's medical school admissions process I would like to provide some guidance. Here's what parents can do to support their aspiring physician.

1. Discuss your child's progress on their terms. Do not push your agenda or constantly ask for updates. The process is stressful, takes an entire year, and is different at each school in terms of deadlines and such. Listen and be supportive and encouraging. The waiting is terrible for many applicants. Your constant asking might be making that worse. If you find yourself micromanaging, this may be an indicator that your progeny lacks the independence required for medicine.

2. Provide your tax information so your child can access financial aid if needed. To qualify for federal aid, all candidates have to provide parental tax information on the Free Application for Federal Student Aid (FAFSA) form. Many schools require it for merit- and need-based aid as well. Usually they only need this information for year one. Candidates who cannot complete their

FAFSA do not get federal aid and may be excluded from institutional aid as well.

3. Help your child reflect, make meaning, nurture identity and purpose, and seek new opportunities. Encourage growth. Listen and reflect back what you hear. Be a sounding board for meaning-making and systems-based thinking/exploration.

4. Offer reassurance and positivity during the preparation and application process. Applicants often get stressed and worried about details and they sometimes need help stepping back and taking in the big picture. It's a perfect role for a parent to offer support by encouraging coping skills and being positive.

5. Participate when asked. There may be a family day, white coat ceremony, and all sorts of celebrations down the road. Be there for those if you are invited.

6. Encourage strong habits of self-discipline, self-care, and time management. A career in medicine is a rigorous path and personal habits of wellness are key. You can offer strong reminders of the importance of maintaining good habits (e.g., balanced eating, adequate rest, exercise, and stress management).

Family Interactions

Students: Please be aware of the way you are treating your parents when you are in public. Treat your parents with respect! If you are rolling your eyes, crossing your arms in frustration, or indicating a poor attitude, we can see that. At one of my schools we host a second-visit event every year and encourage accepted candidates to bring their support team, whomever that may be. Candidates sit with current students, faculty, and staff and chat with them and their guests about the school. A few years ago one of our candidates was seated with her parents and rolled her eyes every time they asked questions. She audibly sighed at their comments and seemed to be unhappy to be there. As a staff, we were puzzled over why she even chose to attend. We were also saddened to see someone so disrespectful to her parents.

Disrespectful behavior of any type reflects very poorly on your candidacy. Remember, many of the people making decisions about your admission are parents ourselves. We see in your behavior the qualities we would *not* want our children to display. Your behavior is indicative of your character. The way you treat your parents demonstrates maturity and integrity. If you do not feel that you can minimize drama when with your parents, avoid bringing them into the equation at all. You appear like a spoiled brat when you disrespect your parents.

How to Be a Good Friend to an Aspiring Physician

Students often tell me that friends are a source of stress in their journey to become doctors. While they are studying for exams and trying to ensure they have covered important preparation areas, their friends often have more free time and do not understand why they cannot go out every weekend. Your friendship and support is crucial to the aspiring doctor in your life. Depending on the aspiring doctor's background, they may need more support from peers and family. Here is how to be a supportive friend.

1. Encourage good coping skills. Help your aspiring doctor learn to manage stress and the inevitable ebbs and flows of life. Getting exercise, eating a healthy diet, and making room for downtime are all positive ways of managing stress and pressure.
2. Find ways to spend time together that accomplish more than one goal. Maybe you meet at the gym and work out together or take a weekly yoga class together. Maybe you plan and cook meals together. Perhaps studying in tandem is a good way to hang out. A weekly joint venture at a local nonprofit as volunteers together might be a great way to stay connected and also use time wisely. Try to be part of the regular support your aspiring doctor friend needs, and understand their time is sometimes limited.

3. Listen and believe. The pathway to medicine can be difficult. When your aspiring doctor calls you to lament the woes of a lab that is not going well or a professor that they feel is sabotaging their dream with a "C" grade, just listen. Yes, they are probably being dramatic and you can tell them that later, but usually they just need your support at that moment. Do your best not to minimize their concerns, but do not engage in the freak-out behavior. Your aspiring doctor will likely have freak-out moments when a B-minus seems like the end of the world. Try to listen and provide perspective.

4. Be mindful of their commitments. The classes your aspiring doctor is taking are very challenging. The premedical science courses may require more time and study intensity than other undergraduate tracks. Understand that your friend may not be able to go out every weekend or party on weeknights. They need sleep and a solid routine. This is just a reality of being premed. They will have fun, but it will likely be scheduled at a time when other demands have subsided for a moment. Be available when that window of opportunity arises. Do not resent your friend if you have to wait until spring break to get some quality time.

5. Understand the time it will take. Your aspiring doctor is pursuing a long-term goal. If they are in undergrad, they will be pursuing admission to medical school, and if they are accepted they will spend four years en route to earning an MD. Following that, they will spend at least three years (and up to seven) in residency. After that they may choose to do additional training in a fellowship program. Throughout these years are important licensing exams, interviews, and application processes. Take some time to learn about their world and be supportive. Be there and be encouraging.

6. Be watchful of their mental health. It is an unfortunate reality that suicide rates are high in the medical profession. Medical students experience anxiety and depression at higher rates, and it often goes unrecognized and untreated. If you see signs that your friend is struggling, encourage them to seek help. Make

sure they know you care and help them follow through with treatment. There are resources at undergraduate schools and medical schools to support mental health.

Your friendship and companionship will be invaluable for the journey.

12

Advice for Advisers

In chapter two, I offered advice for students about engaging with prehealth advisers. Over the years I have met many wonderful advisers who are passionately committed to helping students along their journeys. I have also encountered advisers that I felt were out of touch and that I might caution students about. I have included this chapter for advisers with the hope that it will provide additional guidance to both advisers and students in meeting the demands of preparation both personally and professionally. This chapter might also help volunteer advisers or mentors in providing a larger context that can help provide solid guidance to aspiring physicians. Advising is complex, and there are myriad institutional and individual factors that impact what is offered and how.

I advised students as part of my professional roles at medical schools for many years before becoming a dean, and this experience afforded me the privilege of working with students and seeing their outcomes. I still make time for advising because I know how important it is. I also fully appreciate how challenging it can be. Know that I wholeheartedly appreciate advisers and recognize them as critical to the process.

Meet Students Where They Are

We know that students enter college with varying levels of academic preparation based on their upbringing, high school experience, and access to resources. Colleges should consider this heavily when designing premedical preparation pathways. If your school has only one suggested course track, I would fervently recommend revisiting it and offering more customization. Perhaps there can be one for science majors and one for nonscience majors. Maybe there is a track that includes summers and one that does not. There should be ample opportunities for students to adjust and adapt to life's demands without having to sacrifice performance or well-being. The attrition that we see from students declaring premed at the beginning of college to those that actually apply happens partially because our course tracks are often offered in an inflexible manner.

Students have a higher likelihood of success if they begin the pathway at a level of rigor that fits well with their previous preparation and resources. While many universities do not consider premed attrition a problem, medical schools do. Universities take the attrition as fact and largely expect the typical outcomes, where students are weeded out by Organic Chemistry.[1] Medical schools receive a pool of students and often these students lack diversity or have severe educational disparities that have played out at the college level. These disparities have long-term consequences for the physician workforce. My medical school colleagues and I would ask that undergraduate advising be as holistic as possible.

While premed advisers may have ingrained ideas about certain courses being critical to success in medical school, the truth is that it depends. I have heard advisers say that if a student did poorly in a course at their university it means they will not get into medical school or will do poorly in medical school. While that might be a true assessment for that moment, it is not universally true. Students develop academically at different rates and reach mastery and academic maturity along a spectrum. Medical schools understand this situation, and we even see this trend continuing among our matriculants. While some students bloom early and the academic components come easily, others need a longer runway to fully launch. We look closely at growth and progress, and most medical schools take a holistic approach to admissions. Being honest is important, and being encouraging is equally as critical.

The Sixty-Second Mission Statement

When I advise students I begin with a brief introduction to my approach, akin to a mini-mission statement. I state my commitment to diversifying the profession, my experience working with students over the years, and my acknowledgment of the vast pathways, needs, and backgrounds of students. This helps students understand that while I may not tell them what they want to hear, my honesty is coming from a position of support and belief in them. I tell them that the best advisers are honest, even when it is hard to deliver that honesty. I want to encourage all advisers to develop a personal mission statement and credo about advising and to share that with their students. When you caution students about their performance and what it might mean, they need to know that you are doing your job in being honest about their prospects and opportunities. They also need to know that you are there to support them and encourage their development.

Understand Stereotype Threat

Your identity as an adviser matters, and your identity impacts how students hear your advice. When I hear advisers say, "I treat all my students the same," I cringe. Remember that equity demands that each student receives what they need, not that each student receive the same thing. If we are to address educational disparities passed forward from secondary education, we must attend to meeting students from varying backgrounds where they are.

Jamal and Ms. Hunt

After a discouraging visit from his premed adviser, Jamal, a first year undergrad student, came to my office. We looked at his fall grades, which were a mixture of Bs and Cs. His adviser, Ms. Hunt, had recommended that he take an introductory chemistry course rather than begin general chemistry. In reviewing his grades Ms. Hunt had cautioned Jamal that he needed to do better, especially in his science classes. When I asked Jamal how he felt about the recommendation, he recounted the visit.

She really emphasized my grades being really bad. I explained that it took me half the semester to get my housing straightened out because there was a problem with my financial aid. I was taking the bus and sometimes I missed the first half of class because of the bus schedule. I told her that I get the material—it was just missing those quizzes at the beginning a few times that hurt my grade. I don't think she believed me, like she thinks I'm stupid. She pushed this intro course, which I don't think I need. I asked for information about the doctor shadowing program, but she said that I can't participate in it. I don't know why. It's just like my high school biology teacher all over again.

I listened to Jamal's concerns and offered reassurance that the introductory chemistry class was a good option since it would allow him to settle into his new environment. I emphasized that posting a strong grade point average (GPA) for spring semester would be a good thing, and if it ended up being an easy semester, that's OK. It's not a race, and there are no extra points for doing it faster. I had the information from Ms. Hunt about the shadowing program (she and I were colleagues). I let Jamal know that the program was only open to second year undergrads and above because there's such a high demand. Jamal would definitely be able to sign up in the fall.

After the meeting with Jamal, I called Ms. Hunt. She and I worked well together and she was passionate about supporting students, especially those underrepresented in medicine. So what went wrong here? What was lost in translation? Jamal was a Black man from Chicago's south side pursuing a biology degree and premed at an elite undergraduate university. Ms. Hunt was a middle-aged White woman from the suburbs. Jamal was under stereotype threat. He felt before walking into Ms. Hunt's office that she might not support him. Especially since he had under-performed during the fall semester, he was not going in with confidence. Her honest words were meant to encourage him and ensure he was aware of what he needed to do to be successful, but he heard them differently because of the disconnect between their worlds. She looked like every teacher who had discouraged and discounted him in the past. Ms. Hunt said, "I want you to have time to adjust so that you can begin a stronger performance trend in your science classes." Jamal heard, "I don't think you're very good at science; I think you're stupid." Ms. Hunt said, "The shadowing program is not open to first year students." Jamal heard, "The shadowing program is not open to you."

If you are an adviser, know that your encouragement and advice needs to be as explicit and transparent as possible. Pay attention to the potential for a disconnect and, if you sense it, address it directly. Say what you mean, and say what you do not mean. If you say, "This class is hard," the student might hear it as, "This class is hard for students like you." So instead, say "This class is hard *for every student.*" Take additional steps to make sure that your words and advice are not misinterpreted or misunderstood. "I am saying . . ." and "I am not saying . . ." are important clarifiers if the distance between your identities and worlds is vast. I cannot tell you how many times I have said the same thing as an adviser but it was heard and received differently by a student.

Understand that some students who come from underrepresented backgrounds with few resources have achieved what they have by *not* listening to the advice of those around them. They might not trust easily because the individuals charged with their education may not have lived up to their promises in the past. They may have had to wade through years of naysayers to continue their educational paths. Do not take it personally when your advice is not received well. Change your practice to ensure that it is heard with the love and support you intend.

Tackle Structural Barriers

As the undergraduate student population becomes increasingly diverse, the resources and structures of our universities must adapt.

Take time to understand your student population and address any structural barriers within your control or influence. Consider your office hours and ways that students are able to reach you. Are there additional challenges for working students, commuting students, students with families, veterans, first-generation students, and so on? If you have an ambassador or peer advising program, is it representative and encouraging of all students? Can all students see themselves in the population of peer advisers chosen/endorsed by you? Representation matters.

What are the messages communicated to students through your newsletters, websites, photos, and materials? For whom do these messages resonate and who may not be seeing themselves in your media communications? If there are known barriers related to course sequencing, fees, and committee rules, take on those challenges and work toward equity with your allies and colleagues. I have witnessed advisers change the structure of their letters and committees to be more holistic so as to recognize student development and success. Advisers have advocated for more introductory courses or a change in scheduling that benefited their students. Advisers have also gone out of their way to facilitate access to enrichment and exploration opportunities with the understanding that these opportunities are often not accessible to students with lower levels of social capital because of family of origin.

Be a Personal Trainer, Not a Talent Scout

Advising is becoming more holistic, and I want to emphasize how much medical schools appreciate this development. The role of an adviser can be likened to a personal trainer for fitness. The regimen and recommendations have to be customized and fitted to the athlete. An effective trainer recognizes the varying levels of fitness and the lifestyle aspects that can affect desired outcomes. They might use a variety of strategies to help clients achieve their goals. While group fitness options can be very effective, a personal touch might also be needed. Trainers evaluate their success based on the achieved results of their clients from individual starting points. Clients begin at various stages of health and fitness, and trainers are judged on progress and process.

By contrast, advisers should not have a talent scout mindset. Talent agents look for the best individuals given the characteristics and requirements they have been given from institutions. They are highly selective and only work with a small number of recruits in order to secure a talent slate for the institution. Their job is to discriminate among a large pool of candidates to find the most ideal ones. They measure their success by the number of recruits the institution signs and are not concerned with progress, development, or process. Advisers should not have a gatekeeper or talent scout mindset. Students are best served by advisers who use a coaching and training model.

Vivian and Jade

Early in my career I met Vivian, an expert premed adviser of twenty years. She had shepherded the careers of many students and was a passionate and dedicated advocate. She worked tirelessly to amplify advising strategies that helped students. I learned a lot about helping students through my conversations with her. I called her to ask about a student I had just met—Jade. I knew that Jade was an undergraduate at her university. Jade was a first-generation student from a low-income family and had struggled early in college. She eventually adapted and had been performing well as a neuroscience major since her third semester. Her science GPA was 3.2 and she was heavily considering a postbaccalaureate program for the next two years. I called Vivian to talk through these options, since I was new in my role.

Vivian recommended that Jade extend her undergraduate education by one year in order to take additional upper division, rigorous science courses to improve her GPA and show a solid three years of strong academic achievement. Her university was well regarded and the courses would be looked upon favorably. Jade would have access to full financial aid for her fifth undergraduate year, unlike the postbaccalaureate program, which would only offer limited aid or no aid at all. Jade would not be able to live on campus for another year, but living at home was a viable, financially sound option. Extending the undergraduate time allowed Jade to continue without a gap or the uncertainty of not being admitting to a program following graduation. It would allow Jade to have less institutional transition/uncertainty and continue her strong performance. Vivian helped Jade apply for additional scholarship funds to help cover her fifth year.

Jade did well and applied to medical school the following year after completing more classes to improve her GPA and taking the Medical College Admission Test (MCAT). She was successful in earning a seat in a medical school that was an ideal fit for her goals and needs. This was an exceptionally insightful and creative approach to Jade's situation that took into account her background, resources, and potential. This is the kind of advising that I want to champion—Vivian is an expert premed trainer.

PART V

Gap Years and Reapplying

13
Maximizing a Gap

In years past, most applicants chose to apply during their junior year of undergrad in order to start medical school right after graduation. The senior year of undergrad was busy with applications, interviews, and wrapping up graduation requirements. Nowadays applicants are choosing to take time in between more frequently. Why? More time, new experiences, more preparation, and financial gains are just a few of the reasons someone might opt for a gap. Admissions committees do not view applications differently if a student has taken a gap year. Let's visit some examples.

Jing

Jing worked full-time all during undergrad at a local restaurant. He had a busy schedule with his commitments at work, in the classroom, and on campus. When it came time to study for the Medical College Admission Test (MCAT), Jing knew he did not have enough time with his current schedule. He did not want to rush and take the test without preparing, yet he felt with his current work and course schedule he did not have the time to dedicate to studying. He did not want to let his grades slip trying to do too much at once. Jing decided to do a gap year. In his gap year he studied for the MCAT during May and June, during the hours he usually spent on classes. He took the MCAT in early July and submitted his application around the same time. Jing maintained his job at the restaurant but also was able to seek out more opportunities of interest for his preparation. He shadowed a few physicians in different specialties. He attended research seminars and also increased the hours he spent helping with the youth basketball league at the Boys and Girls Club, where he volunteered regularly.

For Jing a gap year facilitated better balance and a sound approach to the demands of the MCAT and the application cycle. He was realistic about his commitments and set himself up for success by being in charge of his time line. Because Jing had to work, he needed to make adjustments to his approach to make it all happen.

Lizette

Lizette was nearing the end of her junior year and wanted to travel. She had wanted to do study abroad during her junior year, but it didn't work out. She had her sights set on medicine, but she also felt that she needed a break from school. She felt burned out and the thought of continuing school seemed daunting. She applied for a position teaching English in Japan, where all her expenses would be covered to live abroad. She figured she would spend a year teaching and begin medical school after that. Lizette was offered a position and bravely moved the summer following her college graduation. While in Japan she found it difficult to keep up with happenings back home. She realized that her gap year was going to be more than a year because she could not realistically apply from so far away. Plus, Lizette was enjoying her experiences in Japan and wanted to continue teaching. When she was ready to transition back to the United States, Lizette began studying for her MCAT and researching schools. She ended up taking a three-year gap in between undergrad and medical school. The experiences she gained in Japan provided plenty of personal insight and growth for her application. She started school motivated, renewed, and ready to roll.

Whatever you decide to do in your gap, stay focused on personal development and growth. Apply the competitive edge principles (explained in chapter 7) in order to maximize the opportunity a gap year provides. Carefully consider your rationale and be able to explain it to someone. We are supportive of gaps and we understand that there are many reasons for them. What we care about is that you have a plan and continue to develop yourself into a better candidate for medicine.

Kiran

I interviewed Kiran, who mostly worked at Starbucks during his two gap years. I asked him why. He explained that he had a severe health issue toward the end of undergrad and needed health insurance to continue his care. Kiran was offered a solid wage with benefits at Starbucks and took the job. Throughout his time at Starbucks he was able to pay down some debt and save up for medical school, which he thought would set him up for success moving forward. Kiran continued to volunteer and took a few night classes with his tuition benefit to stay fresh on academics. He was able to pause and recover his health before applying. I thought this demonstrated sound judgment and maturity on his part. Kiran also had great insights about coffee and its global influence, effective customer service, and leadership experiences from working at Starbucks.

The key to maximizing a gap year is to have a clear purpose going into it. If you are able to discuss your rationale and explain the benefits, your gap year should serve you well. If your gap year is in the growth zone, better yet. In the end, the journey to medicine is deeply personal and you should take pride in your journey.

Explaining a Gap or Career Change

Over the years I have worked with students who were career-changers with significant gaps between their undergraduate courses and their application. For career-changers, it is important to express why you are leaving your original chosen career for medicine and how you know this is the right choice. You must explain your career-change decision while honoring your first choice, so as not to appear bitter or jaded about what you chose in the first place. It is usually helpful to frame the issue as "wanting more" rather than "dumping my current career."

Khadija

Khadija worked as a nurse in labor and delivery. She absolutely loved being part of the healthcare team and working with patients. As a young adult she had her sights on medicine, but family trauma compelled her to choose a career with more immediate earning potential. She had siblings to support following her mother's death and had to enter the workforce as soon as possible. She chose nursing and finished her BSN in an accelerated program. Khadija had been working for seven years and the thought of being a doctor lingered. Her family was newly stable, and if she did not try to revisit her original dream she knew that she would always wonder "what if." After completing her additional premed courses and taking the MCAT she came to meet with me. We discussed areas of preparation that would make her candidacy well rounded, as she would be applying with students coming out of undergrad. She decided to spend one more year focusing on a research interest and expanding her role at a local clothing donation center. Khadija wrote eloquently about her insights working with patients and what she loved about medicine. She was able to express why she wanted to become a physician and why that role was meaningful to her. With her clinical experience as an anchor and solid preparation, Khadija had several offers for medical school.

For career-changers, it is important to balance your past activities with recent ones. Include some experiences from undergrad years, if relevant, but if the experiences are more than ten years old use careful judgment as to their current relevance. No more than one-third of your experiences should be old. Two-thirds of your experiences should be more current (roughly within the last four to six years). Your letters should certainly be current. Think about it. What your premed committee or professors said about you six years ago is not exactly a recommendation in real time. You have hopefully changed since then. If you are working, please provide a letter from your current employer, if possible. If you are unable to do that, it may help to let us know so that we are not wondering why your current colleagues or supervisors will not endorse you.

Choose your letter writers wisely and provide some guidance to them. The more removed they are from medical education, the more guidance/parameters they may need. I have seen letters that are very off topic and do not address areas of relevance for medicine. I had a former candidate who was leaving a high-level job at an engineering firm. The applicant's letter of recommendation focused heavily on their specific role at the firm and why they were an excellent engineer. It read like a letter for a promotion in engineering. It was less helpful to us in deducing the student's commitment to medicine, potential as a physician, and leadership/people skills. The letter could have focused more on skills that were more transferable or relatable to medicine.

Manuel

Manuel submitted a letter from his eight years of working at a warehouse store. The letter described his character in detail and provided many firsthand examples of why Manuel would be an excellent physician. His supervisor discussed his people skills, altruism, work ethic, ability to learn and adapt, and positive attitude. The letter gave several examples of ways that Manuel demonstrated character, work ethic, and genuine concern for others. The committee weighed this letter very heavily in Manuel's candidacy, despite the fact that it was not from a clinician or professor.

A good rule of thumb for soliciting letter writers is this: Choose people who know you well, not people who have status or titles. You cannot brag about yourself on your application, but your letter writers can certainly heap on the praise. While we may consider whether a letter is from a graduate teaching assistant or a professor, we ultimately care *what* the letter says more than the title of the writer. It is also important to aim for a well-rounded letter packet. This means providing more than one perspective on your candidacy. Schools have varying requirements for letters, usually between three to six total. Some are ultra-specific and some are general. Do your research on school requirements so that you are not caught off guard in the secondary application phase. If all your letters are from professors with whom you've done research, we may wonder about your community or leadership experiences or how you perform in the classroom. Letters should back up the claims you have made in your application. Examine your application and choose letters that will provide testimony on your behalf in those areas. If you have an experience that is a major aspect of your application, do your best to back up that experience with a letter.

14

Advice for Reapplicants

If you are reading this chapter you might be trying to prepare yourself for a worse-case scenario, or you might be pragmatic or pessimistic. It is also possible that you have already received some disappointing news. You are not alone. Remember that more than half (60 percent) of the candidates who apply are not accepted the first time. It's good to prepare for alternative pathways since receiving an offer is never a sure thing. Here is my basic advice for those giving it a go the second (or third or fourth) time around.

Revisit the Growth Zone

The worst thing you can do when not accepted the first time is miss the opportunity for growth and improvement that is lurking within the words of those rejections. Over the years I have worked with countless medical students who were grateful that their first applications were not successful. They will all tell you that at the time it was devastating, but looking back, they later realized it was one of the best things for them and their journey.

It takes about nine months to a year to apply and hear back from schools. The worst thing you can do if you are not successful is submit the exact same application to the same schools with the same supplemental applications and letters that you did the first time around. This is tantamount to insanity. If it did not work the first time, what is going to be different now? Hopefully you continued with your preparation and development and you are able to say what has improved on resubmission. But if not, step back and assess how far you were able to get in the process and what the outcomes were. Gather feedback about your areas of improvement and create an action plan. Do not pressure yourself to get ready to reapply right away. Occasionally someone is especially well prepared and simply applies too late in the cycle, in which case they should still seek feedback advice and update their application before submitting it again.

Analyze Everything

Consider the timing of your application and when your candidacy was complete for consideration at the schools to which you applied. Applying too late can impact the amount of consideration you receive. Most schools employ rolling admissions, so applying in the summer is key. Fall applications get fewer looks.

Review your submissions to schools for supplemental applications. Were your supplemental essays strong? Did you answer the questions specifically for each school? Or did you do too much generic cut and paste? When I review I can tell if someone spent time answering our questions, or if they adapted what they already wrote to try and fit our questions. Also, if there was a suggested character limit and you were way over or way under, that may also have been a small factor.

Consider the number of schools to which you applied. If you did not apply broadly enough, that may have limited your odds. The relationship between the number of schools applied to and the acceptances is positive, but then drops off. There is a sweet spot where you can maximize your odds. Think about it. Each phase results in a reduced number of chances for final selection. If you apply to just eight schools, complete supplemental applications at six of them, get invited to interview at one, then you are down to one chance of getting an offer. Whereas if you apply to fourteen schools, complete applications at twelve of them, and interview at 3, those are higher odds at the end of the process that you could receive an offer. Where you apply is informed, of course, by your personal situation and goals, but a wide net can help maximize your odds of getting a seat.

Consider the mission-alignment of the schools to which you applied against your areas of preparation. If you are applying to a research-intensive medical school you probably should have substantial research experience and deliverables. If the school has a research expectation as part of its curriculum, you should definitely consider whether or not you feel you will be competitive in the admissions process without research experience. Similarly, if the school's mission includes caring for underserved communities, you should have experiences with underserved communities in order to increase your appeal.

Consider your Medical College Admission Test (MCAT) and grade point average (GPA) and the ranges for schools to which you applied. Were you well within ranges for accepted students, or were you below those ranges? Diversity is the name of the game here—and I do not mean your identity. I mean the diversity of schools to which you apply. Choose a few high-profile top schools that are dream schools where you might be reaching, but also include midrange schools where you think you would thrive. Finally, include some backup schools that are also aligned with your preparation areas. Do your homework by researching schools to ensure you have a solid strategy. Only apply to schools that you would like to attend.

Reflect on your letter writers. Are these people who know you well and can specifically comment on your strengths? Did you select individuals who are well aware of your passion for medicine and can testify for you firsthand? If you asked a letter writer because you needed to fill a requisite area, you might have gotten a weaker letter. How confident are you that each of your recommendations is strong and specific? Letters can have an impact on each phase, depending on how schools use them. They can impact review, the interview, and/or final selection.

If you received some interviews but no acceptances, you can feel confident that your written application was compelling enough to merit meeting you in person. So what happened? It could be that you were competitive, but it just wasn't your year. But to make sure that you are better the next time around, seek feedback. Many schools offer a consultation in person or over the phone for reapplicants, but not all do. If you have a mentor or adviser, ask for their feedback as well.

Reflect on your interpersonal skills during your interview day. Were you talkative? Shy? Involved? Withdrawn? How did you feel before, during, and after your interviews? How did you approach your interview preparation? Did you feel well prepared to talk about yourself with a stranger? How do you think you did establishing rapport? Interviewing skills are important because we use them as a proxy for how you will interact with your future classmates and patients. We want to be sure that you are comfortable communicating.

After your interview day, did you communicate your continued interest to the school? Did you follow up with anyone you met? Did you effectively connect with people from the school before, during and after? Most schools have application portals for you to keep them updated on your activities and accomplishments and express continued interest. Use these resources effectively. What about thank-you notes? There is no definitive answer. Some schools give them to committee members at the end of the season only. Some schools forward them to committee members right away. If you are sending a thank-you letter, please make sure that it is genuine. If you are only going through the motions, it isn't likely to help. If you prefer to send a thank-you by email, that's fine. If paper cards are your jam, go with that. One isn't better than the other. Interviewers are usually entering their scores and feedback that day or the following day, so your notes aren't likely to influence their scores.

Seek feedback from trusted, knowledgeable sources who will tell you what you can do to improve. I once had a call with a candidate to advise her about a reapplication and she approached matters beautifully. She started the call explaining her strategy. She had a list of areas that she had identified through self-assessment that needed improvement. For each area she had identified concrete steps she could take to improve. She wanted to use our time verifying that her self-assessment was accurate and that her plans for improvement were well aligned with what she was attempting to address. We talked through each area and I provided feedback on her plans. We made a few modifications. Then she asked a very important question: "Is there anything else in my application that you think needs attention or improvement?" Her approach made it easy to provide constructive feedback. Here are some questions you can use to elicit detailed constructive feedback:

- What is the weakest aspect of my candidacy?
- What is the strongest aspect of my candidacy?
- Was there anything in my application that stood out in a positive way? In a negative way?
- What are some concrete steps I can take to improve my areas of weakness?

Update your application—essays, letters, *everything.*

If you would like us to take the time to carefully evaluate your application, then you should take the time to update it. I can easily pull up your application from a previous cycle and compare it side by side to what you submitted in the current cycle. If I see that you have submitted exactly the same personal statement and answers to our supplemental essay questions, I am disappointed. It clearly sends a message that you did not make the effort to update your materials for my school. I realize many applicants assume that their files are not closely read, and that they think that submitting the same essays won't matter. But what if it does? Why would you go to all the trouble (and expense) of reapplying only to submit the same material and leave that element open for a potentially negative outcome?

Take the time to contact your letter writers, if you are choosing to rely on the same people. Update them on where you are and ask them to submit updated letters of recommendation. They can submit the same letter, but they should update the date so that we know the person still recommends you in real time. If you decide that you need stronger letter writers, take the time to connect with them by phone or in person. Bring a copy of your application and your personal statement. Share your passion and purpose with your letter writers. Let them know why you chose them to write on your behalf. As a letter writer myself, it does help if the student tells me what they would like me to focus on or emphasize in my recommendation. If you are not comfortable initiating these points of contact with your letter writer, ask yourself if this person knows you well enough to recommend you. If you cannot think of at least three people whom you feel can really go to bat for your candidacy in medicine, it's time to head for the growth zone and focus on relationship building and self-development.

Make Reapplying a Strength

Being a reapplicant can demonstrate resilience and help you stand out. It shows determination and investment in your chosen career. It provides an opportunity for you to show a documented growth trajectory. Committees look carefully at improvements that reapplicants have made (or the lack thereof). There are always thousands of reapplicants in the pool each year, so being a reapplicant is not a negative thing. Ensure that you evaluate your candidacy well after an unsuccessful attempt. If you continue to show your growth and commitment, it will shine through the next time around.

15
Finish Lines and Deadlines

Medicine is a fabulous career, but let's be real—it also has many drawbacks. It takes a long time to train and it is years before you begin to specialize in the area of your interest. If you focus your preparation on exploring medicine thoroughly through hands-on experiences outside your comfort zone, you will develop a strong idea of whether it is the right career for you. I am not a dean who discourages anyone's dreams, and I also understand that life goals can be achieved in many different programs and paths. Life can be unpredictable and challenging, and often we must adapt to move forward. If your ultimate goal is to use your gifts to serve others, and the path you choose to get there is highly uncertain and will take at least twelve years, you owe it to yourself to consider other viable avenues to achieve your end goal.

Stacy

Stacy participated in a summer program for premeds during her junior year. She was very set on medicine from day one of college and had not explored other pathways. She experienced difficulty with her Medical College Admission Test (MCAT) and found that time was flying by as she struggled to overcome testing issues and put together an application that was competitive. We met one afternoon and I asked her what she wanted to be able to do with her training. Stacy had worked in patient care as a nurse assistant for a few years and loved being in a clinic.

"I know that I want to pursue primary care. I see myself working in a clinic every day and getting to know my patients. I enjoy the variety of conditions and patients that we see. I just wish there were a fast route where I could train and just do basic patient care every day."

At that point we discussed options—physician assistant (PA) programs seemed a great fit. Stacy had thousands of hours of patient contact, which made her an ideal candidate for a PA program. She had several of the prerequisites already done and could apply while finishing a few of the classes required for PA school. She completed a program in the following two years and passed her licensing exam. Stacy found a more expeditious path to her goal. By staying focused on her vision for her career, she was able to pursue an option that helped her arrive more efficiently.

Give yourself permission to be open to pathways that speak to you. I recommend setting deadlines for yourself and reassessing where you are if those deadlines go by and you have not achieved your goals. You are the navigator of your life. You set the course. Ultimately, it is about finding happiness and balance in a profession that fits well with your skills and values. Be open throughout your preparation. I like to say that if there is anything that you can think of doing that will make you just as happy as medicine (or more happy), do that. I am an admissions dean and, honestly, I have never met a physician who disagreed with this advice. Medicine is a long, expensive training path. What makes it worthwhile is the undeniable truth you possess that it is your calling, to the exclusion of all others. Interrogate your commitment to this calling as actively as you can throughout the process.

Simple Steps to Success for a Career in Medicine and Beyond

I hope this book has eased your worries and given you some practical tips and advice for the journey. I wish for you to feel confident and reassured, as well as more knowledgeable about how to approach your preparation for medicine. It is transformative to become a physician entrusted with the lives and vulnerabilities of your fellow human beings. I want you to know how much the medical education community cares about you. Those of us working in this field love what we do, and we love working with you and seeing your success.

FIRST SIMPLE STEP: BE NICE, WORK HARD, BE SMART

A residency program director once told me that her program looks for the following traits in potential residents: Be nice, work hard, be smart—in that order. This is so simple yet powerful. It doesn't matter how hard you work if you are mean. It isn't helpful that you are smart if you are lazy. If you are kind and willing to work hard, that gets you most of the way. Being smart is more about being willing to learn and put in the work. Many successful people will tell you that they do not consider themselves to be the smartest person in the room, but rather, they are great problem solvers and collaborators and they are confident in their ability to work hard.

SECOND SIMPLE STEP: GET YOUR ADULT ON

I love that your generation made the word "adult" into a verb. In my world it was only a noun. So I offer my very own definition of your newly coined verb: Adulting is parenting yourself. It's pretty simple. All the things parents typically do are now your responsibility. Budgeting and exercising restraint on purchases, cooking meals and grocery shopping, getting your car registration renewed—these are all lovely things we all must do as adults. You will be a happier adult if you also make yourself go to bed at a reasonable hour, eat a balanced diet, exercise regularly, and so on. These are the skills you need to master if you are to be successful in medical school and beyond. Organize your life and your time the way a responsible adult would.

Here is another secret: You are rarely going to feel like adulting. Stop waiting to feel like doing your laundry or studying for that exam. Force yourself to do it! Let's be real. We usually want to watch Netflix all day long, but adulting requires otherwise. Self-discipline is key to success in medicine. You are going to have to tackle tasks that you may find unpleasant in the short term in order to yield long-term gains.

THIRD SIMPLE STEP: ESTABLISH A COMPASS
BY STATING YOUR RULES

Everyone needs a personal credo or rules to live by. Medical training is rigorous, and it is far too easy to lose your way and become jaded, resentful, and depressed. Take time to define what is important to you. Decide what your values are so that you can anchor your preparation experiences in those values. Be conscientious about revisiting your rules periodically. My grandfather left his life rules on a yellow notepad that we found among his things after he passed away. I have them on my wall in my office to remind me of his legacy. Although he was a humble farmer, he reflected on his life and had rules to live by.

Reflection is an amazing tool to continue to bring meaning and purpose to your path. It is important as a premed but remains critical throughout the journey. Reflection and meaning-making are tools of resilience in a sometimes difficult field where suffering and sadness can be daily realities. I am a fan of Futureme.org, where you can send an email to yourself in the future for free. This is a great reflection tool, by the way. I recommend that at least once a year you write a letter to yourself. In your letter reflect how you have grown and changed, write down what you have learned, and express your hopes and dreams for the future. Remind yourself why you chose medicine. Write about patients and experiences that left an impression on you. Repeat this process when you receive your letter each year.

Good Journey

Thanks for letting me share my perspective with you in this book. I am very fortunate to be able to work with students every day and to learn from them. You are the inspiration for this book and are largely the reason I look forward to going to work every day. Although we probably have never met, know that you are a big part of my why and my passion for access, equity, and justice in medicine. I hope that my advice will make your journey a little easier and help you avoid common pitfalls. You now have the tools to thrive and love your premed preparation. My wish is that you will be confident and resilient in pursuing your dreams, even if those dreams happen to change over time. Remember that everything you conquer en route to medicine is ultimately for your future patients. Try to step back and take the long view when life's immediate challenges feel overwhelming. Patients are waiting for a doctor just like you. You are needed. You are important. You are the future of medicine.

Appendix

An Overview of the Journey to Becoming a Physician

Let's start at the beginning with the basics. You might be new to medicine and you might not know what the road map looks like. You might be a parent or friend who would like to get a good sense of what your premed person is about to attempt. As a first-generation college student, I certainly had no idea what the landscape of undergrad, graduate, and professional education entailed. This appendix gives an overview of the journey and includes links to the various resources and services that I've discussed throughout the book.

High School and Undergrad

The journey to medical school begins with courses you take for college credit. For most students this is their undergraduate years. For a few, it might be Advanced Placement (AP) courses taken in high school, or concurrent enrollment courses where college credit is earned in high school. Almost all medical schools require that you earn at least a bachelor's (BS or BA) degree. You can apply while your degree is in progress as long as it is conferred before you begin medical school. There are some BS/MD programs where a student is accepted to medical school conditionally upon beginning a bachelor's degree. You can find those in the Medical School Admission Requirements (MSAR) Online database.[1]

Along with a minimum of a bachelor's degree, you will also need to take the Medical College Admissions Test (MCAT)[2] in order to apply. The MCAT is generally offered January through September. It is not usually offered during the peak of the cycle, which is October to December. When you are ready to apply to allopathic schools that grant doctor of medicine (MD) degrees, you will use the American Medical College Application Service (AMCAS),[3] which can be accessed May 1 and submitted as early as June 1 of each year. Access to the application is free, and applicants pay upon submission of the application. Participating schools specify their own AMCAS deadlines from October through December. It takes a year to apply, so those applying in the cycle that opens in June 2023 would be aiming to start medical school in July/August of 2024. While some graduate or professional programs have multiple start dates, medical schools do not, so the application cycle is annual.

Both the MCAT and AMCAS are owned and operated by the Association of American Medical Colleges (AAMC),[4] which is the nonprofit to which all allopathic medical schools in the United States, Puerto Rico, and Canada that are accredited by the Liaison Committee on Medical Education (LCME)[5] belong. There are two other application services: Texas Medical and Dental Schools Application Service (TMDSAS)[6] and the American Association of Colleges of Osteopathic Medicine Application Service (AACOMAS).[7] The application services are completely separate from one another, and they do not share information. A doctor of osteopathic medicine (DO) degree is an equivalent medical credential to an MD, but the curriculums and emphases of the programs differ between DO and MD. The main difference is that DO trainees learn musculoskeletal manipulation techniques and have greater training on holistic methods and nutrition.[8] Students earning DO degrees also take a different licensing exam.[9] MD and DO programs had separate residency programs in the past, and in 2020 all residency programs integrated to accept both DO and MD applicants, according to the Accreditation Council for Graduate Medical Education.[10]

Upon the submission of an AMCAS application your file will be verified against official transcripts that you submitted separately to AMCAS. This is a part of the service that you are paying for—an expert staff member to review and attest to schools that your transcripts and grades are correctly reported and summarized on your application. You select the schools to which you wish to apply and those schools receive a verified version of your application from AMCAS. There is a cost for the service initially, and an additional cost for each school you choose to send your application to. AMCAS not only ensures that the classes and grades you reported are accurate, it also calculates your grade point average (GPA) for science courses, nonscience courses, and the total. The courses that make up the science GPA are biology, chemistry, physics, and math (BCPM). AMCAS also standardizes the GPA across all submissions by weighting quarter or trimester grades to make them equivalent to semesters. This helps schools compare applicants on different university course schedules more fairly. You may also enter up to fifteen experiences and a personal statement in character-limited fields. AMCAS also has fields for demographic information about you, your childhood setting, your parents, and your family. There is a section where you may indicate if you are disadvantaged and write an explanation.

When schools receive your AMCAS application, they then usually send you a supplemental (or secondary) application. Some schools screen applications before inviting applicants to create a supplemental, and some do not. School-specific information like this is available in the MSAR Online. The supplemental application typically contains school-specific questions and requires an additional fee. This is also the phase where you send your letters of recommendation. Upon receipt of all scores, letters, and requested supplemental materials, a file is complete. At this point most schools employ committees to conduct a review or begin the screening process to decide what happens next.

Every allopathic school requires an in-person interview in order to gain admission. These interviews are invitations extended by admissions committees usually between August and March of the application season. Different formats are used for interviewing, such as one-on-one traditional interviews, multiple mini-interviews, standardized patient interviews, group interviews, or some combination of these methods. Following interviews, the admissions committees eventually report their decisions to applicants based on school-specific processes. The earliest an applicant may hear of a decision is October 15 of the application year.[11] There is a national deadline by which applicants may not hold multiple offers[12] (right now that deadline is April 30). Each school has its own rules about whether you can hold multiple offers past this deadline and when you must declare your chosen school.[13]

Medical School Years One and Two

After enrolling in medical school, students typically spend eighteen to twenty-four months learning basic sciences in the classroom and doctoring skills in simulated and standardized patient (patient actor) situations. There is a licensing exam that allopathic physicians in the United States take that has several phases.[14] The first phase is called United States Medical Licensing Exam (USMLE) Step 1, and it is usually taken after the second year, although some schools have students take it after year three. Step 1 consists of material covered in the first two years of medical school, often called the *preclinical curriculum*. Students are expected to know structures and functions of the human body, organ systems, disease processes, and the associated pharmacological and pathophysiological aspects of treatment.

Medical School Years Three and Four

The next phase is comprised of clerkships/rotations through various specialty areas that typically lasts twenty to twenty-four months.

This is when students get to be a student doctor working with the healthcare team in hospitals and clinics. At the end of the main clerkships of third year, students take Step 2 of the USMLE. There is a *Clinical Skills (CS)* part that is didactic with standardized patients, and a *Clinical Knowledge (CK)* part that is a written exam. The content is based on how to manage patients and various aspects of treating disease in the clinical context.

During the third year of medical school, students begin narrowing down their specialty choice. By the beginning of fourth year, students choose the specific type of medicine they wish to practice: pediatrics, surgery, family medicine, anesthesiology, and so on. During the fourth year students might apply to do rotations at other medical schools in order to better prepare for their specialty. These are called *visiting clerkships or away rotations.* At the beginning of fourth year students apply for residency applications through the Electronic Residency Application Service (ERAS),[15] which is also owned by the AAMC. Again, there are experiences and other standardized data fields for applicants to complete. Similar to medical school, interview invitations are extended to candidates from residency programs. Fourth year students spend time traveling and interviewing for possible residency positions.

In mid-March of every year the National Residency Match Program (NRMP)[16] provides a service to residency programs and applicants that matches them for positions. After interviewing, students submit rank lists of their desired programs in February, and residency programs submit rank lists for their desired candidates as well. The lists all go into a Nobel Prize-winning algorithm and the result is a called a match. The match is a binding employment contract, and students are required to report to their matched program to begin residency around July 1. The shortest a residency program can be is three years, and it can be up to seven, depending on the specialty.

Residency and Beyond

Most programs have trainees take Step 3 of the USMLE following the first year of residency. After passing this final step the licensure process is complete and a physician may practice as a general practitioner, although laws about postgraduate training time vary by state. Upon graduation from residency, physicians may seek board certification from the American Board of Medical Specialties by passing the board exam for their field.[17]

During residency, some doctors wish to apply for additional specialized training through fellowship programs. This might be focusing on a specific organ system, disease, or population for which they are seeking additional training. These programs usually vary in length from one to five years. Following fellowship, a physician may pursue another fellowship or may also wish to seek additional board certifications in their specialty area. Board certifications must be maintained and passed every ten years, typically. In addition to board certification, medical licensure in each state is maintained through Continuing Medical Education (CME) credits required to ensure physicians are staying up to date with their practice.[18] Becoming a physician is truly a lifelong-learning process.

Acknowledgments

This book is the culmination of many years of working with students. Every student with whom I have journeyed has influenced me and helped me grow. I would like to thank my student colleagues for trusting me with their dreams and letting me share in their triumphs and defeats. I consider it my greatest privilege in life to be part of the paths of aspiring physicians.

Thank you to my colleagues in the Association of American Medical Colleges and the Group on Student Affairs. I am beyond fortunate to have you in my life. Over the years we have worked together to enact our vision for medicine. I am indebted to your mentorship, enduring commitment, collaboration, and feedback. Thank you for believing in me and encouraging me.

I would like to express my deep gratitude for my colleagues and students at the University of Utah School of Medicine, Northwestern Feinberg School of Medicine, Loyola University Chicago Stritch School of Medicine, and University of California Riverside School of Medicine.

Thank you to my partner, the one and only Danny Zamarripa, for being my rock. Many times when this book was on the back burner it was you that nudged it forward. Thanks for making me laugh every day and for never growing tired of reviewing what I write. To my three amazing children, thank you for your patience and support of me. Thank you for sharing my passion for teaching and learning, and for always being willing to host a student party at our home.

Thank you to Lisa Banning and the team at Rutgers University Press for giving this book wings.

Notes

Preface

1. https://reflectivemeded.org/2017/02/28/tough-love-for-your-personal
-statement-advice-from-a-medical-school-dean/.

1. Premed Basics

1. AMCAS Application Guide. https://aamc-orange.global.ssl.fastly.net
/production/media/filer_public/b2/23/b223c482-8ba3-44dd-bb1c
-8835ac84f3e6/2020amcasapplicantguide-060419.pdf.
2. National Student Clearinghouse Research Center, Time to Degree.
https://nscresearchcenter.org/signaturereport11/#targetText
=Enrolled%20Time%20to%20Degree,5.1%20academic%20
years%2C%20on%20average.
3. Flexner Report. http://archive.carnegiefoundation.org/pdfs/elibrary
/Carnegie_Flexner_Report.pdf.
4. Prepare for the MCAT Exam. https://students-residents.aamc.org
/applying-medical-school/taking-mcat-exam/prepare-mcat-exam/.
5. U.S. MCAT Calendar, Scheduling Deadlines, and Score Release
Dates. https://students-residents.aamc.org/applying-medical-school
/article/mcat-testing-calendar-score-release-dates/.

2. Advice for First-Generation Students

1. https://students-residents.aamc.org/applying-medical-school/article
/amcas-letter-service-advisors-and-other-letter-aut/.

3.   Advice for Minoritized Students

1. Thomas Neville Bonner, *Iconoclast: Abraham Flexner and a Life in Learning* (Baltimore: Johns Hopkins University Press, 2002).

2. Sunshine Nakae, *The Backgrounds and Outcomes of Allopathic Medical School Applicants: Exploring Stratification and Inequality* (dissertation, Loyola University Chicago, 2014), 1294.

3. American Medical Association, "Medical Education and Its Recognition by the Rich," *Journal of the American Medical Association* 37 (July–December 1901): 32; American Medical Association, "An Overcrowded Profession: The Cause and the Remedy," *Journal of the American Medical Association* 37 (July–December 1901): 775–776.

4. Claude Steele, *Whistling Vivaldi: And Other Clues to How Stereotypes Affect Us* (New York: W. W. Norton, 2010).

5. Lisa R. Grimm, Benjamin Lewis, W. Todd Maddox, and Arthur B. Markman, "Stereotype Fit Effects for Golf Putting Nonexperts," *Sport, Exercise, and Performance Psychology* 5, no. 1 (2016): 39–51. http://dx.doi.org/10.1037/spy0000047.

6. J. Stone, C. I. Lynch, M. Sjomeling, and J. M. Darley, "Stereotype Threat Effects on Black and White Athletic Performance," *Journal of Personality and Social Psychology* 77, no. 6 (1999): 1213–1227. http://dx.doi.org/10.1037/0022-3514.77.6.1213.

7. R. P. Brown and E. A. Day, "The Difference Isn't Black and White: Stereotype Threat and the Race Gap on Raven's Advanced Progressive Matrices," *Journal of Applied Psychology* 91, no. 4 (July 2006): 979–985.

4.   Advice for Undocumented Students

Thank you Yadira Ortiz, Denisse Rojas Marquez, Erick Leyva, and Rico Oregon for reviewing this chapter.

1. Special thanks to the Pre-Health Dreamers (PHDreamers.org) network, for its constant collaboration and the many opportunities provided for me to serve as an ally over the years.

2. Sunny Nakae, Denisse Rojas Marquez, Isha Marina Di Bartolo, and Raquel Rodriguez, "Considerations for Residency Programs

Regarding Accepting Undocumented Students Who Are DACA Recipients," *Academic Medicine* 92, no. 11 (2017): 1549–1554. doi: 10.1097/ACM.0000000000001731.

3. "What Is AB540?" https://ab540.com/.

4. Medical School Admissions Requirements. https://students-residents.aamc.org/applying-medical-school/applying-medical-school-process/medical-school-admission-requirements/.

5. California Senate Bill 1159. https://leginfo.legislature.ca.gov/faces/billTextClient.xhtml?bill_id=201320140SB1159.

8. The Inside Scoop on Strategy and Maximizing Mission Fit

1. Medical School Admission Requirements, "Search Institutions." https://apps.aamc.org/msar-ui/#/landing.

2. AAMC Fee Assistance Program. https://students-residents.aamc.org/applying-medical-school/applying-medical-school-process/fee-assistance-program/.

3. https://www.usmle.org/.

4. https://reflectivemeded.org/2017/02/28/tough-love-for-your-personal-statement-advice-from-a-medical-school-dean/.

5. https://students-residents.aamc.org/applying-medical-school/article/application-and-acceptance-protocols-applicants/.

6. https://students-residents.aamc.org/applying-medical-school/article/application-and-acceptance-protocols-admission-off/.

7. See the Liaison Committee on Medical Education, standard 10.7, *Functions and Structure of a Medical School.* http://lcme.org/.

9. Understand the Graduate/Professional School Context

1. https://www.aamc.org/data-reports/students-residents/report/facts.

2. https://www.aamc.org/system/files/2019-10/2019_FACTS_Table_A-16.pdf.

3. https://www.aamc.org/system/files/2020-04/2019_FACTS_Table_A-23_0.pdf.

10. Professionalism and People Skills in a Digital Era

1. Maxine A. Papadakis, Arianne Teherani, Mary A. Banach, Timothy R. Knettler, Susan L. Rattner, David T. Stern, J. Jon Veloski, and Carol S. Hodgson, "Disciplinary Action by Medical Boards and Prior Behavior in Medical School," *New England Journal of Medicine* 353 (2005): 2673–2682. doi: 10.1056/NEJMsa052596.

11. Advice for Parents and Friends

1. Laura McKenna, "The Ethos of the Overinvolved Parent," *The Atlantic*, May 18, 2017.

12. Advice for Advisers

1. Karen Lovecchio and Lauren Dundes, "Premed Survival: Understanding the Culling Process in Premedical Undergraduate Education," *Academic Medicine*: 77, no. 7 (2002): 719–724.

Appendix

1. https://students-residents.aamc.org/applying-medical-school/applying -medical-school-process/medical-school-admission-requirements/.
2. https://students-residents.aamc.org/applying-medical-school/taking -mcat-exam/.
3. https://students-residents.aamc.org/applying-medical-school/applying -medical-school-process/applying-medical-school-amcas/.
4. https://www.aamc.org.
5. http://lcme.org/.
6. https://www.tmdsas.com/.
7. https://www.aacom.org/become-a-doctor/how-to-apply-to -osteopathic-medical-college.
8. https://choosedo.org/why-consider-a-career-in-osteopathic-medicine/.
9. https://choosedo.org/board-examinations-and-licensure/.

10. https://acgme.org/What-We-Do/Accreditation/Single-GME
-Accreditation-System.

11. https://students-residents.aamc.org/applying-medical-school/article
/application-and-acceptance-protocols-admission-off/.

12. https://students-residents.aamc.org/applying-medical-school/article
/application-and-acceptance-protocols-applicants/.

13. https://students-residents.aamc.org/applying-medical-school/article
/amcas-choosing-your-medical-school-tool/.

14. https://www.usmle.org/.

15. https://students-residents.aamc.org/applying-residency/applying
-residencies-eras/.

16. https://www.nrmp.org/.

17. https://www.abms.org/board-certification/.

18. https://www.medscape.org/public/staterequirements.

Index

connections, personal, 63–64, 109, 152
context: advisers providing, 132; graduate/professional school, in application strategy, 99–107
continuing medical education (CME), 143–144, 166
coping skills, 34, 128, 129
copycat syndrome, 58
coursework, undergraduate: customization of, 5–10, 22, 132–133; pace of, 3–12, 133, 138–139
critical-thinking skills, 64–70
curiosity, 65, 72
customer service, 60–61, 112–113, 145. *See also* employment
customization: of advising, 137–139; of premed course pathways, 5–10, 22, 132–133

Dana, story of, 62–63
Danesh, story of, 29–30
date, earliest acceptance, 76
deadlines: AMCAS, 162; for decisions and declarations, 164; for financial aid, 93; for prehealth committees, 21; in professionalism, 114; self-set, for career decisions, 155–156; for supplemental applications, 78–79
debt, consideration of, 54, 95–96
Deferred Action for Childhood Arrivals (DACA), 36–37, 39–40. *See also* citizenship status; undocumented students
demographics, 103–104, 163
development, academic, 133, 149–150
development, personal: advisers in, 137; campus resources in, 26; of character, in professionalism, 111–112; in a competitive edge, 72; in maximizing gap years, 144–145; meaningful experiences in, 55–57; in reapplying, 149–150, 153; in rejection, 105–106
disability community, 63
discernment of career choice, 49–54
discouragement: from advisers, 18,

24–25, 134–136; stereotype threat in, 134–136
disparities, educational, 133, 134–136
diversification of undergraduate majors, 12
diversity: advisers in improving, 133, 136–137; and equity in education, xii; of first-generation students, 14–15; of schools, in reapplication strategy, 151
Dream Centers, 39–40
DREAMers. *See* Deferred Action for Childhood Arrivals (DACA)

Electronic Residency Application Service (ERAS), 165
e-mail addresses, professionalism in, 111–112
embellishment of applications, 57–58
Emergency Medical Technician (EMT), 34
Emilia, story of, 18–19
empathy, demonstrating in personal statement, 87
employment: authorization for residency, 36; for first-generation students, 13–14; during gap years, 143–144, 145; during medical school, 41; in personal growth and people skills, 60–61, 112–113
engagement: academic, in pacing of coursework, 11–12; community, in a competitive edge, 63–64; in outside activities in creating support, 34; in professionalism, 116–118; in real life medicine, 54; in systems-based thinking, 68–69
enrollment management, 92–93, 103–107
entitlement, 99–100, 106–107
equity, 134–136, 137
essays. *See* personal statements
Evelyn, story of, 123–124
exclusionary practices in allopathic medicine, 27
executive function skills, 10, 82

inclusion of minoritized students, 27–28
independence: in competitive edge,
62–63; Dana, 62–63; for first-
generation students, 15; independent
learning guide, 66; in learning style,
Cameron, 96–97; Lizette, 144–145;
and parental involvement, 123–126, 127
inexperience, acceptance of, 28–30
intentionality: in the application
process, 82; in career choice, 50, 54; in
choosing experiences for growth,
55–56; in making connections, 109; in
organization of application materials,
82; in pacing of premed, 3; in seeking
advice, 19–20; in self-care, 35
interviews: analyzing, in reapplying,
151–152; cell phone use during, 118;
checklist mindset in, 55–56, 57–58,
60–61; gap years in, 145; in the
graduate/professional school context,
103; immigration status in, 39;
interpersonal demeanor in, 23;
parents attending, 125; personal
statements in achieving, 86, 89–90;
professionalism and people skills in,
108–109, 114, 118–119; for residencies,
165; self-advocacy through, 90;
systems-webs in preparing for, 65,
68–69; thank you notes following, 152

Jade and Vivian, story of, 138–139
Jamal and Ms. Hunt, story of, 134–136
James, story of, 51–52
Jared, story of, 69–70
Jerica, story of, 43–44
Jing, story of, 143–144
journey overview, 161–166
judgment: gap years demonstrating, 145;
in professionalism, 116, 118–119

Khadija, story of, 146
Kiran, story of, 145

leadership, 70–71, 72, 145, 148
leave of absence from medical school, 41
letters of intent, 91–92

letters of recommendation: for career
changers, 146–148; letter service,
AMCAS, 21; in pacing of coursework, 11–12; by parents and family
members, 126–127; from prehealth
committees, 20, 21–22, 23; in
reapplying, 149–150, 151, 153–154
LGBTQ students: Albert, 33; Ari,
10–11; Cameron, 96–97; Cassie, 59;
Lizette, 144–145; Lydia, 34–35.
See also identity
Liaison Committee on Medical
Education (LCME), 162
licensure and licensing exams, 40, 81,
164–166
listeners: friends as, 130; on support
teams, 33–34
Lizette, story of, 144–145
low grade point average (GPA), 52
Lydia, story of, 34–35

major, choice of, 12
market competition for students,
103–104
Marnie, story of, 23
mastery, academic, 133
maturity, 11–12, 53, 119, 133, 145
meaning-making: in career success, 158;
and the checklist mindset, 56, 58; in a
competitive edge, 62–63, 65, 68–69;
in gap years, 146; parents supporting
process of, 128; in rejection, 105–107
Medical College Admissions Test
(MCAT): in admissions/acceptance,
81; analyzing, in reapplying, 151; in
application delays, 80; in applying for
admission, 162; average scores on, in
acceptance rates, 100–101; expiration
of scores, 9; during gap years,
143–144; in pace of coursework, 7–9,
11–12; premed coursework influenced
by, 7–9; reduced fees for, 77; timing
of, 8, 11–12, 80, 143; tips on, 79–81;
voiding scores on, 79. *See also*
American Medical Colleges,
Association of (AAMC)

About the Author

SUNNY NAKAE, MSW, PHD, began her career in medical education in 2001 as a program coordinator for diversity and community outreach programs at the University of Utah School of Medicine. She fell in love with medical students and the intersection of communities and medical education. Through her outreach role, Dr. Nakae began to work with aspiring doctors on all facets of preparation. She served in leadership positions in both diversity and admissions committees through the Group on Student Affairs (GSA) at the Association of American Medical Colleges (AAMC). Early in her career Dr. Nakae moved to Chicago, where she directed the Office of Diversity at the Feinberg School of Medicine at Northwestern University and continued to expand her role as an adviser, student advocate, and admissions committee member.

Dr. Nakae completed her doctorate in 2014 with a study of stratification and inequality in allopathic medicine by examining admissions outcomes. She became the Assistant Dean for Admissions, Recruitment and Student Life at the Loyola University Chicago Stritch School of Medicine later that year. There, she designed and implemented innovative holistic review tools aligned with the school's mission. Dr. Nakae has continued her leadership within the GSA at AAMC by serving on the Advancing Holistic Review Advisory Committee.

In early 2019, Dr. Nakae transitioned to the University of California, Riverside School of Medicine as Associate Dean for Student Affairs and Clinical Associate Professor of Social Medicine, Population and Public Health. Her current role involves admissions, pipeline programs, and the care and keeping of medical students. Her research and scholarship continues to focus on access and equity in medical education and healthcare.

Dr. Nakae earned her bachelor's degree in Human Development and Family Studies and a master's degree in Social Work at the University of Utah. She completed her doctorate at Loyola University Chicago. She lives in Riverside, California, with her partner and their three children. You can find her on Twitter @ DrNakae and on YouTube, where she gives a weekly pep talk for medical students called "Dean Nakae's Med School Minute." She can be reached at premedprepadvice@gmail.com.

Printed and bound by CPI Group (UK) Ltd, Croydon, CR0 4YY

27/10/2024

14580229-0001